"I lost 30 pounds in 30 days just from juicing."

— *Camille, secretary, United States*

"I have clear skin. No more acne!"

— *Jenna, aerobics instructor, Australia*

"I lost 40 pounds in eight months!"

— *Diane, teacher, United States*

"Forty-three pounds lost so far in three months."

— *Sarah, United States*

"I am fighting my cancer, thanks to the Earth Diet recipes."

— *Mark, accountant, United Kingdom*

"I've been drinking one green juice and one lemon juice a day for the past seven days, and have lost a half pound a day effortlessly. Love it."

— *Pat, United States*

"My diabetes has improved, and this is the most free I've ever felt in my body."

— *Carly, aspiring dancer, United States*

"I have replaced my antidepressant medication with juicing. Thank God! Thank you for the Earth Diet recipes. They are delicious."

— *Eddie, event director, United States*

"I have been using the Earth Diet recipes since March 2012. My eyesight has improved so I don't need as strong contact lenses. I have lost 30 pounds and been able to keep it off consistently. I now juice every day. I make Superfood Kale Salad every other day."

— *Kate, social worker, United States*

"I want to commend Liana on the Earth Diet. More than 50 of my patients have used her recipes and are feeling better, slimming down, and making healthier choices for themselves and their families!"

— *Dr. Thomas Ianniello, United States*

"I had pityriasis rosea and doctors said there was no cure. Eight days on the Earth Diet recipes and it was completely gone."

— *Cate, IT manager, United States*

"I made a lot of the Earth Diet recipes, and since I've started eating this food, I am beating my cancer. Two of my tumors have gone. If you just want to get healthier and feel awesome, you need to check this book out. Seriously."

— *Marie, United States*

"Dear Earth Diet, I have been using your recipes for three weeks now. Within the first five days, my stomach issues, as well as my chronic heartburn, cleared up. I am no longer bloated and my energy has skyrocketed. I'm steadily dropping weight, too. I love, love, love the recipes from the Earth Diet and have gotten compliments at work. Thank you for changing my life."

— *Vickie, United States*

"The Earth Diet recipes provide the solution for people to feel better, to live better, and to be healthier. Since I found the Earth Diet six months ago, I have lost 20 pounds, gained more energy, and become more of the man I want to be. I love my body and I am very grateful for your recipes. My favorite thing about the Earth Diet is being encouraged to eat raw chocolate every day."

— *Noah Loin, Raw Chocolate Man*

"I was scared for my life. Now I have it back thanks to the Earth Diet recipes!"

— *Lawrence, business owner, Canada*

"I lost 40 pounds in three months gradually and consistently while putting so much goodness into my body. I ate raw cheesecake and chocolate, ice cream made with nuts, and things sweetened with honey and maple syrup instead of refined sugars. I forced myself to juice every day, and then found I enjoyed it. I never felt deprived, just so nourished with good foods that actually taste good and that I feel no guilt about eating."

— *Christine, massage therapist, United States*

"I love this totally natural lifestyle and the simple concept of eating the cleanest possible. I have never felt so healthy, thanks to the Earth Diet recipes."

— *Laura, nutritionist, United States*

"I broke my addiction to refined sugars. I now enjoy real sweets—raw chocolates made with cacao and desserts that I feel good about—and have lost weight. It's really quite unbelievable. I have lost 15 kilos and I'm still going. I am excited to wake up in the morning because I get to eat chocolate."

— *Sandy, Australia*

"The juice and lemon water each day got me. Totally makes sense! I feel more balanced, and my life is becoming more and more enjoyable the better I feel."

— *Nadia, mother, Philippines*

"In a world filled with quick fixes and fad diets, it is so refreshing to see someone step up to inspire and teach people to eat healthy and live more congruently, the way nature intended."

— *Dr. Billy Chow, chiropractor and wellness mentor*

"Eating directly from nature—as nature intended—is the only way to eat. If only everyone could realize the long-term benefits of a healthy lifestyle. After all, a healthy body is the key to a healthy mind."

— *Eric Merola, director of* Burzynski: Cancer Is Serious Business

"Since starting the Earth Diet eight months ago, I have lost 30 pounds and kept it off. I had eczema and it's not completely clear yet, but I definitely experience less irritation and it is gradually healing. The Earth Diet is the ultimate all-inclusive guide to clean, conscious eating. As I have gradually adapted the principles of this amazing lifestyle into my day-to-day life, an incredible transformation of my health has occurred, and my sense of balance has been restored. The process of health is ongoing. Once you realize that, the pressure is off! The Earth Diet meets you at your level and supplies you with the proper tools. The rest is up to you!"

— *Salvatore, health coach, United States*

"I healed myself of testicular cancer with juicing, coffee enemas, and switching to a plant-based lifestyle."

— *Chris, entrepreneur, United States*

"I was told that herpes cannot be cured. I did the Earth Diet for three months and then tested negative. I did the Earth Diet Detox with juicing and mostly raw vegan recipes and have not had an outbreak in 11 months. I am free of herpes. I am not embarrassed to tell you this; I am just grateful it is out of my life. I am convinced it is gone for good if I keep up this lifestyle. It makes sense to me that when my body is fed healthy foods, my immune system can beat any sickness."

— *Matt, finances, United Kingdom*

"I did the juice fast and in four months lost 45 pounds. I have been able to keep it off, and I am who I am supposed to be today . . . and it doesn't stop here. My life is forever changed, and I can only improve from here on out."

— *Donna, nanny, United States*

"I love the simplicity of the Earth Diet. It's the way we were meant to eat, and if we could start from scratch, we'd find everything has been created for us to give our bodies exactly what they need."

— *Marilynn Pridham, fitness model and personal trainer*

"The Earth Diet helped me transform my life in so many ways. I was overweight and I lost 15 kilos, and my skin and all my school grades have improved *heaps*! I juiced my mum some beets and made her some raw chocolate peanut butter balls on Mother's Day. She couldn't believe that the chocolate she was eating was actually *good* for you! Also, being 15 years old, I used to think that I had to be super skinny and starve myself. Reading what you say about inner being and just being yourself has taken me so far. I have really changed my outlook on life. I can't thank you enough."

—*Jade C., student, Australia*

"I have been juicing daily ever since starting the Earth Diet, and the three major differences I notice are an increase in energy, feeling really good, and a boost of confidence."

—*Lisa, sales rep, United States*

"I have never felt better than I do being on the Earth Diet. This is a great way to get back to feeling healthy and fit at the same time. I have lost ten pounds so far, and absolutely love how I feel. Thank you, Liana, for introducing this to me while I was in New York."

—*Melissa, United States*

"After I was diagnosed with adrenal fatigue in June last year, I became more aware of what I was eating and putting on my skin. Now I am super conscious of what I eat and put on my skin so I can get well. The Earth Diet is a wonderful reference. I love having a name for what I eat and how I live!"

—*TJ, United States*

"I have to thank you for the Earth Diet, as I was addicted to chocolate. Before I would easily eat over half a block of chocolate every night, and now I buy less, or no, shop-bought chocolate. I have been making my own with cacao from your recipe, and some nights I have been able to go without any chocolate, where I would never have been able to do that in the past. I'm starting finally to feel free from that huge sugar craving I've always had, so thanks again."

—*Jade, Australia*

**To read stories of people who have used the Earth Diet and see their transformation photos, visit TheEarthDiet.com/BookGift.**

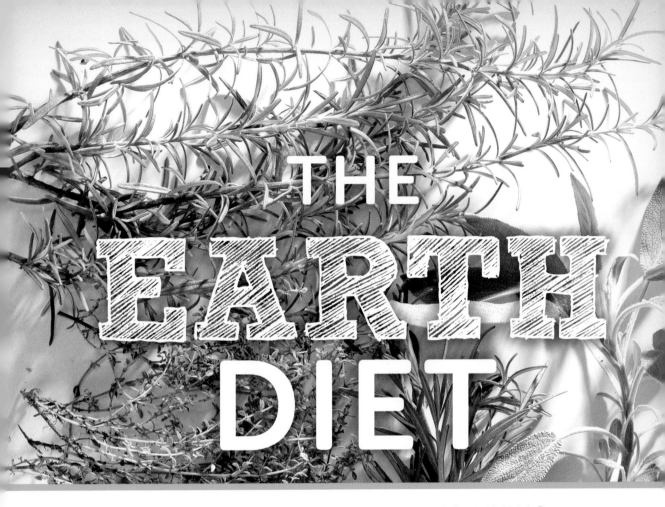

# THE EARTH DIET

## YOUR COMPLETE GUIDE TO LIVING USING EARTH'S NATURAL INGREDIENTS

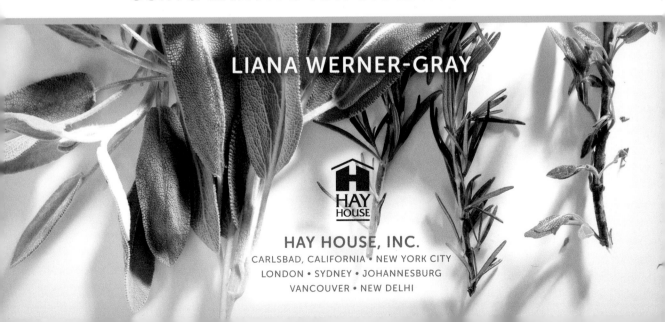

### LIANA WERNER-GRAY

HAY
HOUSE

## HAY HOUSE, INC.

CARLSBAD, CALIFORNIA • NEW YORK CITY
LONDON • SYDNEY • JOHANNESBURG
VANCOUVER • NEW DELHI

Published and distributed in the United States by: Hay House, Inc.: www.hayhouse.com® • Published and distributed in Australia by: Hay House Australia Pty. Ltd.: www.hayhouse.com.au • Published and distributed in the United Kingdom by: Hay House UK, Ltd.: www.hayhouse.co.uk • Published and distributed in the Republic of South Africa by: Hay House SA (Pty), Ltd.: www.hayhouse.co.za • Distributed in Canada by: Raincoast Books: www.raincoast.com • Published in India by: Hay House Publishers India: www.hayhouse.co.in

**Cover and interior design:** Georgia Rucker

**Interior photos:** Original photography by Allen Owens/Limoncello Productions except for the following:
p. vii and 23: topseller/Shutterstock.com; p. viii: Mazzzur/Shutterstock.com; p. xi and throughout (texture) Asya Alexandrova/Shutterstock.com; p. xii: Wang Song/Shutterstock.com; pp. xviii and xix courtesy of Liana Werner-Gray; p. xviii and xix: Edward Fielding/Shutterstock.com; p. xx: optimarc/Shutterstock.com; p 6: ©iStock.com/wragg; p. 7: ©iStock.com/sbayram; p. 8: Lubava/Shutterstock.com; p. 9: ©iStock.com/redmal; p. 11: Nikitin Mikhail/Shutterstock.com; p. 12: Tim UR/Shutterstock.com; p. 34: matin/Shutterstock.com; p. 40: ©iStock.com/Oktay Ortakcioglu; p. 56: Volosina/Shutterstock.com; p. 57: MidoSemsem/Shutterstock.com; p. 58: SOMMAI/Shutterstock.com; p. 59: Volosina/Shutterstock.com; p. 60: Dmitrij Skorobogatov/Shutterstock.com; p. 61: marekuliasz/Shutterstock.com; p. 63: tehcheesiong/Shutterstock.com; p. 64: Peter Zijlstra/Shutterstock.com; p. 65: Banner/Shutterstock.com; p. 66: Asya Alexandrova/Shutterstock.com; p. 66: Valentyn Volkov/Shutterstock.com; p. 67: Nattika/Shutterstock.com; p. 68: KIM NGUYEN/Shutterstock.com; p. 69: Andrey Starostin/Shutterstock.com; p. 73: Elena Moiseeva/Shutterstock.com; p. 79: Diana Taliun/Shutterstock.com; p. 83: Paulista/Shutterstock.com; p. 85: Diana Taliun/Shutterstock.com; p. 88: Kesu/Shutterstock.com; p. 92: matin/Shutterstock.com; p. 99: Dionisvera/Shutterstock.com; p. 100: Valentina Razumova/Shutterstock.com; p. 110: Dionisvera/Shutterstock.com; p. 111: draconus/Shutterstock.com; p. 117: ©iStock.com/marekuliasz; p. 118: sevenke/Shutterstock.com; p. 122: Imageman/Shutterstock.com; p. 125: Andrey Starostin/Shutterstock.com; p. 126: Coprid/Shutterstock.com; p. 130: Deep OV/Shutterstock.com; p. 135: leungchopan/Shuttterstock.com; p. 136: Peter Zijlstra/Shutterstock.com; p. 138: SOMMAI/Shutterstock.com; p. 140: Sally Scott/Shutterstock.com; p. 142: 123rf.com/viktoriya shvydkova; p. 144: Scisetti Alfio/Shutterstock.com; p. 150: hsagencia/Shutterstock.com; p. 153: jocic/Shutterstock.com; p. 154: Nattika/Shutterstock.com; p. 157: Dancestrokes/Shutterstock.com; p. 168: graph/Shutterstock.com; p. 170: kesipun/Shutterstock.com; p. 174: mylisa/Shutterstock.com; p. 176: mexrix/Shutterstock.com

Library of Congress Cataloging-in-Publication Data

Werner-Gray, Liana.
  The earth diet : your complete guide to living using earth's natural ingredients / Liana Werner-Gray. -- 1st edition.
      pages cm
  Includes index.
  ISBN 978-1-4019-4497-1 (tradepaper : alk. paper)  1.  Natural foods--Therapeutic use.  2.  Cooking (Natural foods) 3.  Self-care, Health. I. Title.
  RM237.55.W47 2014
  613.2--dc23
                                    2013035834

Tradepaper ISBN: 978-1-4019-4497-1

10  9  8  7  6  5  4  3
1st edition, October 2014

PRINTED IN THE UNITED STATES OF AMERICA

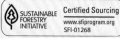

SUSTAINABLE FORESTRY INITIATIVE Certified Sourcing www.sfiprogram.org SFI-01268

SFI label applies to text stock only

This book is for every human being who wants to **live a healthier life.**

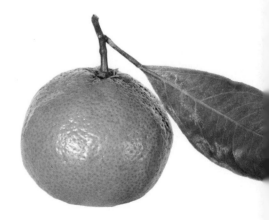

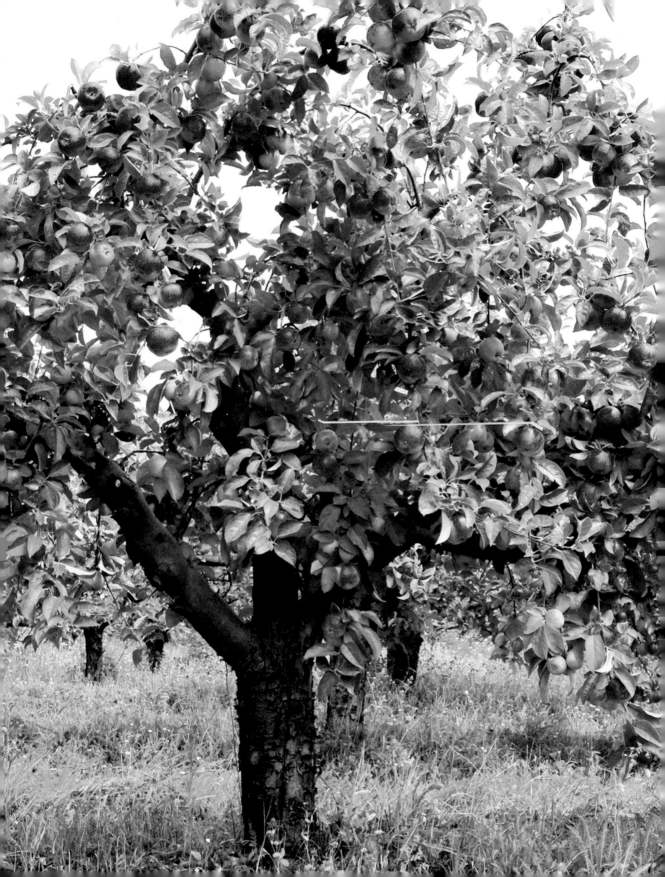

# CONTENTS

# PART III: The Earth Diet Guides

# Author's Note

This book is based on the author's own personal experience, conclusions, beliefs, and opinions and is not intended to diagnose, treat, or prevent any illness or condition. Use this book entirely at your own risk and responsibility. As with all diets, please consult your preferred medical professional before starting the Earth Diet. The book contains general information only. Please note that:

- Information provided in this book is not intended as a substitute for advice from a registered physician or other health-care professional.

- Information is intended as a guide only. Readers should always conduct their own research and consult with their preferred medical practitioner before making any decisions about matters concerning their health.

While the author has endeavored to ensure that all information provided in this book is accurate and up-to-date, the author takes no responsibility for any error or omission relating to this information. She will not be liable for any injury, illness, loss, or damage suffered by you or others through your use of the information provided in this book. The author, publisher, and or distributors of this book are not responsible for adverse effects or consequences resulting from any suggestions from this book.

You must not rely on the information in this book as an alternative to medical advice from your doctor or other professional health-care provider. If you have any specific questions about any medical matter, you should consult your doctor or other professional health-care provider. If you think you may be suffering from any medical condition, you should seek immediate medical attention. You should never delay seeking medical advice, disregard medical advice, or discontinue medical treatment because of information in this book.

That being said, always listen to and trust your own advice.

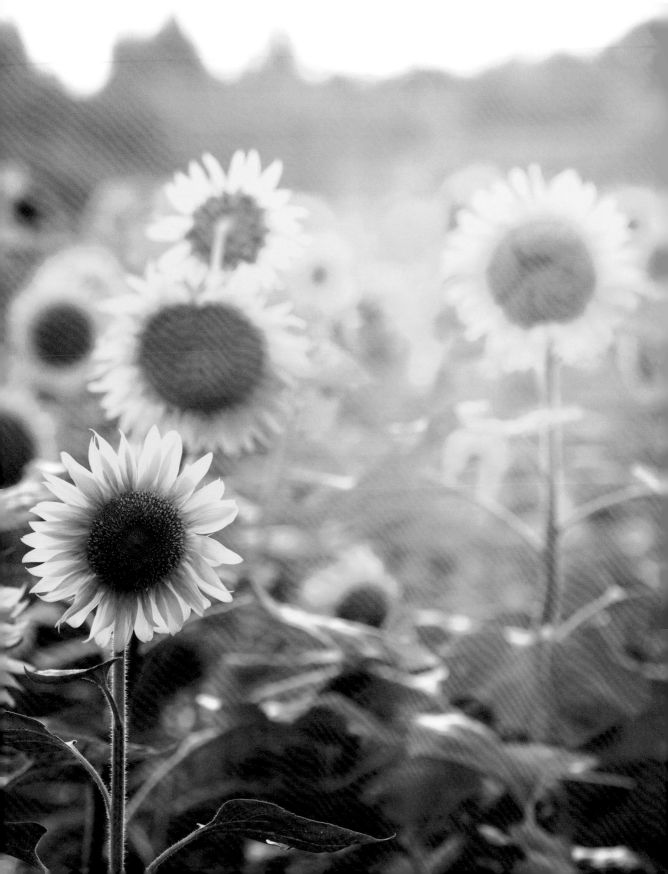

# "I want to feel my life while I'm in it."

— Meryl Streep

My name is Liana Werner-Gray. Here is a long story made short: I was really, really sick, so I changed my lifestyle to be more natural and Earth-friendly, using the recipes in this book, and was healed. Today I lead a healthy, energetic life and help other people to do the same by sharing my recipes and nutritional information with them.

Of course there was a lot to it, and I'll share the details of my journey. I was born and raised in Australia, and I excelled at school. Mostly I got A's and was often awarded achievements and distinctions in math, English, science, sports, and the arts. I broke school records. At nine, I won a competition to get a storybook published that was shelved in the Darwin Library. I was a healthy, happy, confident kid and ate well-balanced meals that my parents provided.

But when I graduated high school and moved away from home, something shifted. I took control of my food choices—and I didn't make good ones. From ages 17 to 21, I ate processed junk food literally every day: sugary candy and greasy hamburgers, pizza, and chips.

After a while, it felt like my body was severely lacking energy. I was tired and gaining weight and confused. Knowing how bad my junk-food diet was for me, I tried to stop.

I wasn't at all happy with my choices. Every day for five years I promised myself, *This is the last day. Tomorrow I will start over and be healthy—and I won't eat junk food ever again.* That's when I realized I was addicted. Like a drug, junk food gave me a temporary high. I liked *that,* but not what came after it.

Although I enjoyed the taste of what I was eating, it was having a terrible effect on my body. Because of how I ate, my life wasn't going where I wanted it to. I felt completely unfulfilled and out of touch with my purpose. I was neither able to achieve my immediate goals, nor was I living my dream life.

Occasionally I would starve myself for a couple of days to try balance out the amount of calories I had taken in from overeating. Then I'd binge again because I was so hungry— my poor body!

When I was alone, a sense of anxious discomfort and heaviness would come over me. I'd wrestle with thoughts of going to get a pizza or hamburger. After a while I'd give in and then be so disappointed with myself. I'd think, *I blew it! The day is already ruined! I might as well eat more.*

I didn't know it at the time, but some would consider this an eating disorder. I'm sharing this part of my story with you so that if you're going through something similar, you'll know that no matter how bad or stuck you may feel right now, there is a way out. If I could make the changes I'll be describing later, you can, too. Eating properly helps. It shifts everything—and faster than you might imagine right now. When you begin nourishing yourself, your body is restored to balance, and you create a new relationship with yourself that rests on an unmovable foundation.

But at the time, because I was ashamed, I hid the truth of how I was eating from my friends and family, and my confidence diminished. Hiding left me feeling even worse about my body and myself. I knew this lifestyle wasn't right for me and hoped that someday it would change. I honestly thought that one lucky day I'd just wake up, and my cravings magically would be gone.

Meanwhile it felt like I was waiting for my life to begin. I had dreams of becoming a professional actress and a film producer, of traveling the world—and of having a healthy, strong, fit, and flexible body—but it was like there was an obstacle in my path that I couldn't remove. Of course, now I understand that although I was eating a lot, I was malnourished; thus my brain and my body weren't functioning properly. My dreams were out of reach because, for one thing, my junk-food habit was costing me a lot of money. I also had cellulite and bloating, and my energy and confidence were too low for me to pursue my career ambitions. I remember often having the thought, *This isn't it yet.* But the more pain and suffering I experienced, the more I wondered, *Why do I keep doing this to myself? Why am I eating foods with no nutritional value?*

So there I was, watching my life go by, feeling unhappy, and dragging myself around in a tired, sluggish body. All the while, I was so sad that I was living such an unfulfilled life—and I was only in my early 20s!

## My Wake-Up Call

Then I got sick. One day, I was at a concert with friends, and all of a sudden it felt like something in my neck popped. A mini-explosion. I reached up to find out what was going on and felt a lump like a swollen gland. I figured it would go away on its own if I got enough rest, drank lots of water and ginger tea, and ate garlic. This is what I normally do when I catch a cold. But over the next two weeks, that lump got bigger and harder. Ultimately it reached the size of a golf ball, and I realized I should get it checked out.

I got multiple opinions. One medical doctor told me that I was having an allergic reaction to cats. Then I went to a naturopathic doctor who sent me to the hospital for a biopsy. They took out a piece of the lump for testing, and I had to wait a week for the results. I remember that when I went back, I sat in the waiting room feeling really upset about my situation and trying to make deals with the Universe. You know the kind I mean: *Please, please, please . . . I promise. If you make this okay, I'll never deprive my body again!* I wasn't surprised by my condition because I knew I hadn't treated my body well. Through my choices, I was preventing myself from feeling good. I was saddened that I had let things get to this point.

The nurse told me to go in and talk to the doctor. He told me, "The good news is that it isn't cancer. The bad news is that a lump of precancerous cells have come together in your lymphatic system. You have these choices. We can either wait to see what happens; we can do surgery and remove it; or we can start you on a treatment of radiation right now, which would make it shrink."

I knew that being in the hospital getting diagnosed with a tumor at 21 was far too young. I hated the idea of radiation. So right then and there I decided I would turn the experience into a positive, healing event. This was going to be my opportunity to end my struggle with junk-food cravings once and for all and to transform my life and body. I got how serious my condition was.

Getting the tumor was a blessing in disguise. It gave me the extra push I needed to make a real change. It brought me, finally, to the day when I thought, *This is it!* On that day, sitting in the hospital listening to the doctor, I told myself, *I will not and cannot live another day like I am.* What the change would look and feel like was actually something I had been fantasizing about and planning for a couple of years. I knew that I wanted to feel inner peace, go back to my roots, and reconnect with the Earth.

I felt something that I imagine might be close to the fear and sadness that many people feel when getting a diagnosis of cancer. But I chose to walk out of the hospital that day believing it was possible that I could heal myself by modifying my lifestyle and diet rather than by undergoing conventional treatments that might be toxic. I would discover that I was not alone in this. More and more people around the world have been making similar decisions. I'm not trying to set rules for anyone else's behavior; I'm just sharing my story. Each of us has to follow our own instincts when it comes to healing, and this decision was right for me.

## The Transformation

I started doing research, meeting with doctors who prescribe natural treatments, and reading books that confirmed my belief that I could treat myself with the power of nature. Knowing that other people were having success healing themselves naturally gave me the confidence to do it. It was finally time to restore my body with nutrition and love. It was time to embrace a consistently healthy lifestyle.

I won't lie to you. It was hard in the beginning. At the time, I felt drained. I was at rock bottom. The tumor was stopping the flow of energy through me, and I felt sore and ugly. My body was expelling toxins. It was swollen, inflamed, and achy. It hurt to swallow and to talk, and my skin and eyes were slightly yellow. Feeling very sick, I was nonetheless sure I could improve my situation by putting proper nutrients into my body. I began drinking fresh vegetable juices a couple of times a day, along with herbal teas and soups. Physically, I felt even worse for at least a month. My body was weak and tired, as if I had the flu, because I was detoxifying. Emotionally, I felt relieved that I wasn't going to be stuck in my vicious cycle of consuming junk foods anymore.

I know the exact moment my deepest healing happened. During that awful first month, I was lying in bed one night and thought, *Now I know what it feels like to have my health taken away from me. I can either get worse and die from this tumor, or I can completely heal and be free of it.* The next thought was that I preferred to heal and be free of it.

It was a moment of pure clarity. It was obvious that I was already going in the direction of healing.

Some sort of heavy energy lifted off me then. Everything shifted in that instant.

Then I thought, *I'll keep doing what I'm doing and just wait for my body to catch up.* From that day, the tumor began dissolving.

My junk-food cravings lessened over the weeks that followed, although they still weren't entirely gone. To satisfy those urges, I created my own healthy alternative recipes for things like chocolate, hamburgers, pizza, and chips. With a little creativity, I found that I could keep enjoying my favorite tastes and textures, while also packing my meals with nutrients.

Sure enough, within three months of adopting this natural lifestyle I had entirely self-healed the tumor in my throat. In the process, I learned that Earth's natural ingredients and thinking good thoughts are the perfect healing combination. I am living proof! I am now healthier than ever.

Due to following the Earth Diet lifestyle for several years, my life has been transformed in every way. I look better, I feel better, I have more energy, I've lost excess weight, my immune system is strong, I'm confident and assured, and my mind is sharp because my body is fueled daily by life-giving foods.

Maintaining good health is now easier for me. I love and appreciate my body more than ever. I am relieved no longer to be addicted to junk food. I now fuel my body with nourishing foods that give me the energy I need to live a great and active life. I eat food every day that tastes good and incorporates the most natural, healthy ingredients nature has to offer. I am a more positive, aware, and peaceful person. I am actively pursuing my dreams. Although I still encounter obstacles on occasion, food is not one of them.

The Earth Diet has given me my life back.

## Sharing My Journey

My diagnosis came in January. Three and a half months later, in early April, the growth in my throat was gone, and I felt better. But I was very afraid that I might slip back into my old habits. One of the first steps I took to reinforce my new lifestyle was to start writing a blog called "The Earth Diet" with an intention to post once a day for 365 days straight to establish consistently healthy habits. The people who read it held me accountable. I mentioned it on Facebook, and slowly more and more people began to follow my progress.

Around the world, indigenous people on different continents have lived off the land without technology and by harvesting what Earth provides. In Australia, the Aboriginals live healthy lives even in one of the harshest desert environments on the planet. If they could do so, I was sure I could do it also where I lived in the city of Brisbane, taking advantage of all the modern conveniences and terrific natural ingredients at my disposal.

Where did I get my determination to pursue a course of natural healing? From watching elderly people since I was very young, I saw that they usually gained weight and ultimately died of an illness like cancer. I thought this was the norm until my classmates and I were taken on a school excursion to the outback, near where my family lived in the town of Alice Springs. Aboriginal elders we met there showed us how to survive off the land with no machinery or technology. I wanted to be like them. I saw how they gathered their food from different trees and bushes, and from hunting wild animals, and how they put it all together to create nutritious, good-tasting meals.

The Aboriginals I knew as a child lived a long time and rarely got sick. They only ate whole, organic foods from the earth and their physical health reflected this. They lived in lean, fit, flexible bodies rather than being overweight and burdened by diabetes and other diseases. They were proof that our health does not have to decline as we get older and, in fact, it can even get better. From them I learned that we have control over our well-being because we have control over our thoughts and what goes into our bodies. I wanted to be like the Aboriginal elders I admired.

As I pursued this goal, people started reading my blog, following it regularly, and e-mailing me about my posts, saying that they had experienced the same vicious cycle with junk foods as I had and how thankful they were that I was sharing my experience with them. Their support and encouragement uplifted me. In a spirit of community, I shared the new recipes I was creating, and my readers loved them!

After my initial year of blogging, I decided to continue and chose to dedicate my life to the earth and to sharing the good news of the healing power of the Earth Diet recipes. I kept doing a lot of research and testing, and took workshops and classes with experts around the world. I wrote and self-published an early edition of *The Earth Diet* with the help of many of the experts whose work I had studied and read about. Very quickly, the lifestyle I was developing—pumping the body full of nutrients from nourishing whole foods—came to be known by many as the simplest way to lose weight and heal.

When I started to help other people eat right, I saw how fast most of them gained vitality, raised their energy, and improved their overall health. I became even more fascinated by nature's simple, clean ingredients and the role of food in our health. Soon I started leading my own workshops and giving seminars on the Earth Diet, and these got positive feedback. I heard from more people who were losing weight with little or no effort, just from enjoying healthy, great-tasting juices, smoothies, and meals based on the recipes I was providing. I also heard from those who had improved or reversed health conditions related to their lifestyle—conditions like diabetes, cancer, bloating and other digestive issues, acne, psoriasis, eczema, heart disease, and more. From their results, I came to the conclusion that anything and everything that's ailing in the body can be improved by proper nutrition. That philosophy is the basis of the Earth Diet. I have now made it my mission in life to spread my knowledge worldwide.

## My Mother's Healing

The Earth Diet has extraordinary personal meaning for me. In 2012, my mother was diagnosed with advanced breast cancer. Determined to help her cure herself with the same methods I used, I created a program for her that included daily juicing and meals made from Earth Diet recipes. Following this plan, her health was restored in a rapid four months. That solidified my commitment to my teaching. I realized I had found my calling and purpose in life.

I am here to spread the message that it is possible to self-heal from anything, even the most serious diseases, and achieve optimal wellness through natural means. I am a messenger of hope.

I know not everybody will be physically cured of their serious, life-threatening diseases by modifying their diet and lifestyle alone, but I always hope they can. Despite any prognosis, I believe that everybody can get at least somewhat better if they rely upon the gifts that nature has provided for us.

I am so grateful for the healing my mother and I have experienced. It is my mission to ensure that as many people as possible learn about the wonders of nature and what a natural diet can accomplish. I love the hugs I receive from grateful people I meet who have achieved their fitness and health goals with my support.

## Life Is Good!

Health is a choice we make from moment to moment. We do not have to suffer from food addictions and illnesses our entire lives. Best of all, we can be free of the burden of eating guilt- and regret-inducing foods! I am living proof that we have the choice and power to change our experience. I am pursuing the path where my body is consistently healthy and disease free. I found a way to nourish my body with good-tasting, nutritious food. Now it's your turn.

Here are some of the results people are commonly achieving with the Earth Diet.

- Weight loss
- Clearer and more radiant skin
- Feeling good
- Effortlessly toning and building muscle
- Breaking addictions and vicious cycles with food
- Unmovable self-love and self-respect
- Raised confidence
- Increased energy
- A better relationship with food

Here is a photo of my mother on the day after she was diagnosed with advanced breast cancer in both breasts. This was the day she started juicing. In this shot, she is drinking her first-ever juice! Fortunately, my mum is healthy and cancer free to this day. The exact healing protocol she followed can be found on my website: TheEarthDiet.com/BookGift.

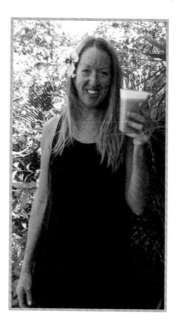

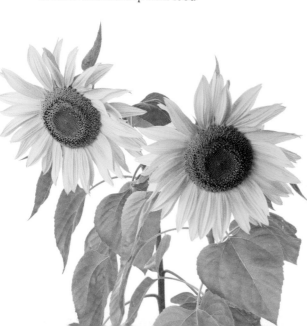

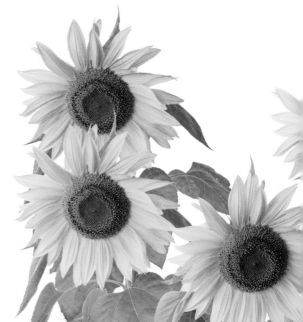

In this book, you'll be introduced to recipes for great-tasting juices, milkshakes, smoothies, raw and cooked vegan dishes, healthy dishes for meat eaters, condiments, desserts, and teas with healing benefits. I'll share tips and techniques for natural body care and self-healing. You'll also find guidelines for weight loss, clear skin, juice cleansing, building muscle, boosting your immunity, and even indulging your sweet tooth while still receiving optimal nutrition. The beauty of the Earth Diet is it can be adapted to you and your lifestyle and needs.

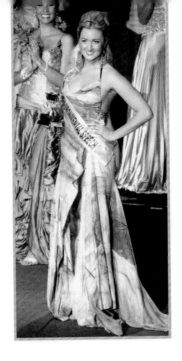

The Earth Diet gave me my life back, so that now I have an energetic, good-feeling body to live inside, instead of a sick-feeling, burdened body. My hope is for you to experience the same. I want to give back to you all for buying this book. To say thank you, I have included some free gifts for you at TheEarthDiet.com/BookGift.

With love,

Liana Werner-Gray

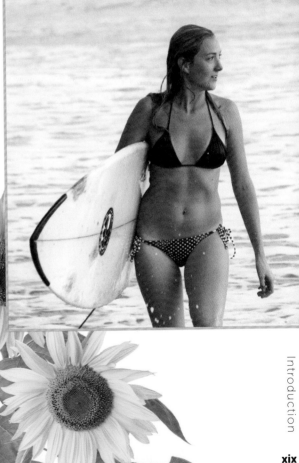

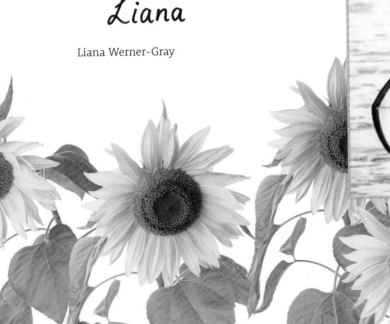

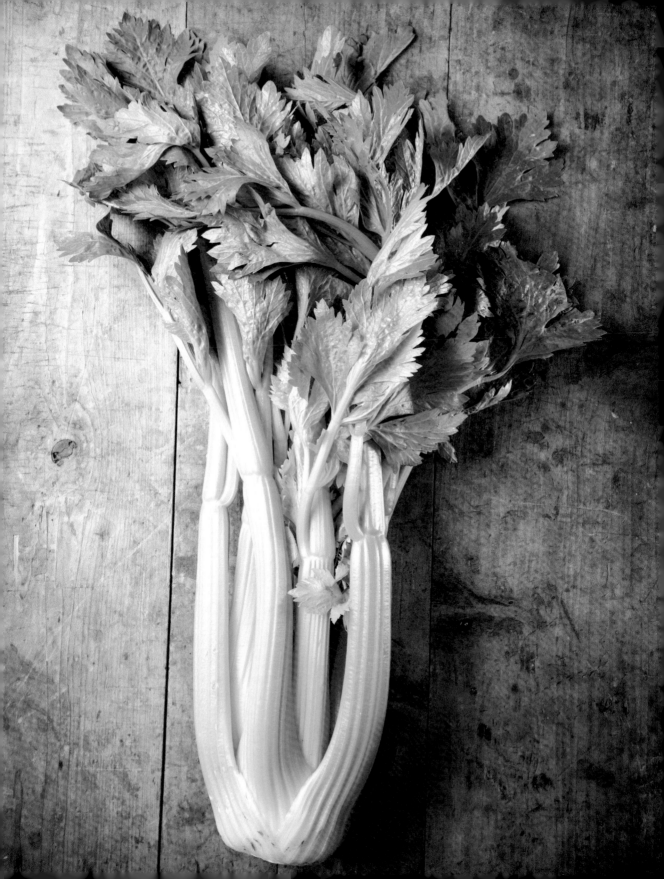

# PART I

# Why the Earth Diet?

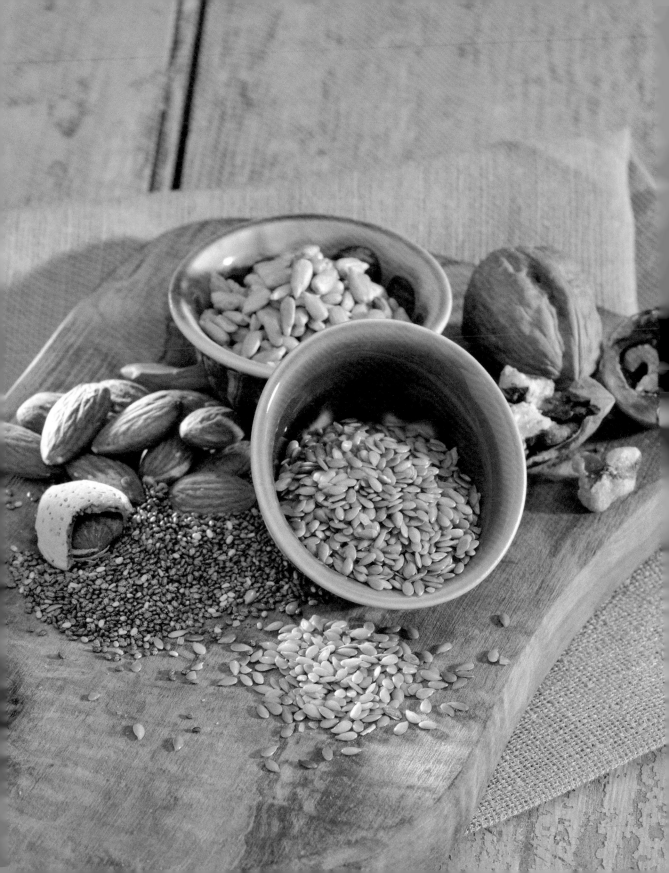

# CHAPTER 1

# The Earth Diet Basics

## The Earth provides us with everything we need.

Is the Earth Diet a hard lifestyle? No, it is the simplest. Why? Because we focus on eating only what is provided for us by nature.

We live the Earth Diet lifestyle by adhering to simple guidelines in the areas of:

**FOOD CHOICES.** We eat ingredients that are naturally provided by the Earth. We avoid processed foods and incorporate whole, organic foods.

**OUR CHOICE OF SERVICES.** We patronize businesses that use ingredients naturally provided by the Earth, and we purchase services from providers that incorporate "green" practices into their businesses, like using organic products and sustainable energy.

**OUR CHOICE OF PRODUCTS.** We understand that with every purchase we make, we are voting, so we purchase products that use ingredients naturally provided by the earth. By supporting local farmers and buying foods that are in season, local, and organic, and otherwise voting *yes* to Earth-friendly products,

these will become more accessible to us and more affordable.

The Earth Diet foods are appropriate for people of all ages and genders. In general, it is safe to follow these guidelines because the diet is not restrictive in terms of calories—it's not a fast. It is nutrient dense, and actually protects you from ingesting toxic chemicals. Remember always to consult with your health-care provider, however, if you have any doubt about your condition or suspect you need to limit certain food items based on your unique circumstances, which might include allergies. People with weakened immunities, heart disease, or cancer; those who are about to have or have just had surgery; and pregnant or nursing women may want to be sure they are receiving the right amount and kind of nourishment, and therefore they should also communicate with an expert.

One of the beauties of eating according to the Earth Diet guidelines is that we are taking in so many nutrients, any deficiencies we might have previously experienced disappear.

By eating this way, our nutritional needs are easily met. We're naturally consuming a well-balanced variety of foods. In just one fruit juice or vegetable juice, for example, you'll usually get a big dose of vitamins A and C.

The Earth Diet is designed for every type of eater from the exclusively raw vegan to the vegan who eats cooked food to the meat eater. Rather than judge other people's food choices, I advise that you concentrate on making your own choices the best ones for you. People who have specific allergies can easily modify the recipes. A short explanation of modifications is offered in Chapter 4.

You can expect many good things to happen to you when you live the Earth Diet lifestyle. Eating whole foods from the Earth that are chemical free strengthens the immune system and increases energy. When the body is energized, we feel good and are better able to fight off sickness and cope with stress. The modern world holds an incredible amount of pressure—to be perfect, to move quickly, to be successful, and so on—and this approach is a key preventive strategy for wellness and mental health. The Earth Diet recipes are designed to make us feel good, while providing our bodies with optimal nutrition! Often the body returns to its ideal weight when we eat this way, so we may even lose excess pounds.

Why do the Earth Diet? To live your healthiest life possible. It is crucial to get sufficient nutrition on a daily basis. Through proper nutrition a lot can be achieved: fitness, mental clarity, and a sense of confidence and personal empowerment. I believe that any negative health condition can be improved, and I hear from people all the time describing their specific gains. When they begin using the Earth Diet, they tell me that they are getting relief from ailments that include

everything from diabetes and cancer to acne, depression, and candida imbalances. In my experience, the Earth Diet can upgrade the health of every person because we are what we eat, and if we eat well, we are well. The body is built from the food we eat, the air we breathe, the emotions we feel, and the thoughts we think.

The Earth Diet improves the quality of our lives by helping us feel and look good. Imagine how much better your life would be if you felt at ease and energized the vast majority of the time. What would be different? When I altered my lifestyle, I dropped weight and my energy soared. As I described in the Introduction, I healed a tumor the size of a golf ball in three months from changing my diet; reducing stress through meditation, relaxation, massage, acupuncture, and other natural methods; and practicing positive thinking and self-love. I had been going, going, going, and eating junk food along the way. By attuning myself to the needs of my body, I understood more of what it needed—intuitively I knew whether I should take a hot bath or get particular nutrients, like vitamin C. I also altered the pace at which I was living. I reprogrammed some negative thoughts. I used to cope with my stress by eating junk food, and it was a huge relief to let that habit go. It was awesome to discover I was in charge of my health and choices.

All of us can benefit from eating highly nutritious foods. Every human body needs to receive a wide variety of vitamins, minerals, phytonutrients, and amino acids to sustain itself and function properly. Raw, whole, plant-based foods—meaning those that are consumed in their natural, unrefined state—provide us with the enzymes and life-force energy we need to survive and thrive. And it's really a no-brainer to avoid eating and drinking anything that has toxic chemicals in it. I mean, come on, which would you prefer, a plump, juicy orange grown with or without pesticides? Would you rather eat a happy chicken that lived its life running around freely in a field or one that lived a miserable life cramped in a cage, was fed genetically modified (GMO) grains, and got injected with hormones and antibiotics?

Toxic foods drain us of energy and have the potential to cause a lot of health issues. Foods that come to us relatively intact have more nutrients. Their value hasn't been depleted by how they are harvested and the machinery used for sterilizing, shipping, and packaging. We're going to take more benefits from an organic apple grown from an heirloom seed that we pluck from a tree ourselves and eat right on the spot, than from eating a chemically sprayed, GMO apple that was shipped across the country via plane and then was waxed before being placed in the supermarket bin for two weeks before we find it. If our bodies are consuming a lot of toxic material along with our food, we are working hard to digest fiber and protein and getting limited energy in return. This leads to weight gain, sluggishness, and ill health.

You'll be happy to know that you can avoid all this by using the Earth Diet, which is extremely flexible. Using the recipes, you can tailor your food choices around your lifestyle goals, such as to lose or gain weight healthfully, to gain muscle if you're an athlete, to improve your moods, and more. This lifestyle has you feeling better as soon as your next meal—your next guilt-free meal! It has you living with increased energy and mental clarity immediately. One of my friends even told me her eyesight improved noticeably within a couple of days. She now wears "weaker" glasses.

## The Earth Diet Principles

Practically speaking, the Earth Diet is simple. This lifestyle replaces all processed ingredients with what the earth naturally provides and emphasizes positive, environmentally sustainable behaviors. Earth Diet foods are mostly whole, some raw, and a majority are plant-based. Let's define a couple of those terms.

**WHOLE FOODS** are unprocessed—meaning, unaltered—types of produce, like an apple, an avocado, or a bunch of parsley. They are foods in their most natural state. Whole foods have been proven to provide our bodies with more nutrition than processed foods, as all of their nutrients are intact.

In culinary vernacular, **RAW FOODS** are uncooked or dehydrated at temperatures below 105°F. By virtue of the guidelines for the Earth Diet, you'll find yourself eating raw the majority of the time without needing to think about it. A salad is raw. A juice is raw. A nut milk or fruit smoothie is raw. When you eat an apple or a carrot or a handful of blueberries, that's raw, too. In this book, you'll find delicious recipes for raw vegan main dishes, as well as **HYBRIDS**, dishes that are partially raw and partially cooked.

### SIMPLE TIPS FOR ADDING MORE RAW FOOD TO YOUR DIET:

- Eat raw with every cooked meal. For example, French Fries can be eaten with Green Salad.
- If you make a soup or curry, rice or pasta, serve it with fresh raw herbs like parsley and cilantro, and add cucumber, sprouts, and avocado.

**HERE ARE THE BASICS.**

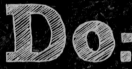

# Do:

- Eat real food made from Earth's natural ingredients. If the Earth doesn't grow it, don't use it!

- Use organic produce as much as possible.

- Juice daily for enhanced cellular nutrition.

- Grow your own produce when possible.

- Use produce that is locally grown as much as possible.

- Use seasonal produce as much as possible.

- Before every meal, ask, "Am I getting the nutrition I need from this?"

- Eat intelligently. Rely on your wisdom and natural instincts.

- Eat a majority of raw, plant-based foods: fruits, vegetables, nuts, and seeds.

- Nourish your body regularly. Eat small meals spread out by two to three hours.

- Tend toward simpler meals, such as "mono" meals (consisting of one food only) or Earth Diet recipes that have only three to five ingredients.

- Prepare and cook your food yourself as often as possible.

- Drink two to three liters of clean, filtered water every day.

- Drink Lemon Water (see p. 100) upon rising every day to detoxify and alkalize your body. This also gives your body a quick infusion of antioxidant vitamin C, folate, and potassium.

- Eat food that makes you feel happy.

- If you choose to eat meat, use organic meat from animals that range free, are given non-GMO feed grown without pesticides, and are raised without growth hormones and antibiotics.

- Use fish that is wild caught rather than farm raised.

- Use eggs from chickens that range free, are given non-GMO feed grown without pesticides, and are raised without growth hormones and antibiotics.

- Eat organic chocolate occasionally, if you like dessert!

- Practice daily affirmations, such as: *I deserve superb health* and *I love myself and eat the best food from Mother Earth that nourishes my body.*

- Use natural skin products to avoid chemicals. If you can't eat something, don't put it on your skin.

- Exercise regularly.

- Live the practice of nutrients in, toxins out.

- Eat when you're feeling relaxed.

- Share food with people you love.

- Eat outdoors, surrounded by nature, as often as you can.

- Define your health dreams and know they are possible.

- Commit to the Earth Diet one day at a time, one meal at a time, one choice at a time.

- Choose to feel good.

- Choose to feel good again and again.

- Remember that every journey takes place one step at a time.

- Do the best you can.

- Realize how good a person you really are.

- Know that health is an ongoing process.

- Be kind to yourself.

- Have fun.

# Don't Eat:

- Refined sugar or aspartame. Instead, for sweetness use dates, fruits, raw honey, maple syrup, cane sugar, pure agave, and stevia.

- Refined flour (bleached white flour is the worst). Instead, use whole-wheat flour. For gluten-free options use buckwheat flour, rice flour, oat flour, almond flour, and other nut flours.

- Gluten (unless you have a healthy digestive system).

- Processed white table salt. Instead use clean salts that provide the body with minerals, such as Himalayan salt and sea salt.

- Canola oil and generic "vegetable" oil. Instead use oils that are especially nourishing for the body, like flaxseed oil, extra-virgin coconut oil, extra-virgin olive oil, and avocado oil.

- Foods, like margarine, that contain partially hydrogenated fats and trans fats.

- Dairy (unless it is organic and raw, from healthy cows). Instead, use nut milk and seed milk. If you are going to consume cow, sheep, or goat's milk, the best kind comes from local farmers whose animals are roaming freely and eating natural, organic feed and grass.

- Non-organic meat.

- Genetically modified (GMO) foods.

- Foods containing corn or corn syrup—the majority of corn is GMO.

- Soy (except organic in very small quantities if you do choose to have it in your life). The majority of soy is GMO.

- Foods that contain chemical additives such as preservatives, fillers, flavorings, colorings, MSG, and stabilizers.

- Highly processed foods.

- Foods with dozens of ingredients. On the Earth Diet, we aim to keep things simple.

- Fast food (the new type of organic fast food is an exception).

- Fat-free foods.

- Foods that have ingredients you cannot pronounce: for example, synthetic foods that list their ingredients as numbers.

- Packaged foods that are fast, cheap, easy, and fake.

- Irradiated and microwaved foods. Microwaves change the molecular structure of food, leaving it with very little nutritional value—or even none.[1] Also, the foods people typically cook in their microwave ovens are frozen, convenience foods, which tend to be highly processed.

- Foods that have come from far away, like the other side of the globe.

- Frozen foods—some organic frozen fruits are an exception.

- Canned goods. New organic products in BPA-free cans are an exception.

The Earth Diet is not a diet in the traditional sense of restrictions we place upon ourselves and being deprived of our favorite tastes and foods to achieve the bodies and health we desire. That's not the case here. In this book, the term *diet* simply refers to a way of eating. The Earth Diet could also be called the Earth Lifestyle because it is a lifestyle choice. You simply eat what you want when you want as long as you are hungry and the food is nutritious. The rule is that you use Earth's natural, organic ingredients to make great tasting foods.

Some people think healthy food tastes gross. This is the opposite of my experience and of many others when they begin using the Earth Diet recipes. In the beginning, your taste buds and body might be used to refined sugars and other processed foods. But gradually, as you cleanse those from your system, you will naturally gravitate to healthier options and *love* the taste of them. There is no better fulfillment than eating delicious-tasting foods that also leave us feeling so nourished and energized. Food that makes us feel tired and sick afterward sucks. I used to get excited about processed chocolate, ice cream, and hamburgers. Now, believe it or not, they make my stomach turn—and thank goodness I crave these toxic foods less and less—but it took me years to achieve this.

Now I get excited about Earth Diet chocolate, vegan ice cream, and my home-made burgers. I enjoy what Gwyneth Paltrow says in her book *It's All Good*: "Most importantly, no matter what you want or need to cut out, for whatever reason, mealtimes should always feel happy. Not like a punishment. If I've learned anything, it's that it's all a process. 'Falling off' your plan is part of it, not a reason to beat yourself up. It takes time to make these changes. It's all good." She also quotes Dr. Habib Sadeghi, an osteopathic physician, who agrees that healthy food can and must excite us: "A lot of people think great flavor is an afterthought when it comes to 'healthy' food, but if we are to be fully nourished by food, it needs to taste wonderful. Food must be a pleasure-filled, spiritual experience. God gave us taste buds for a reason!"

You'll be glad to know that on the Earth Diet you are not required to count calories—unless you really want to. When you eat natural foods, over time the body is restored to its natural and ideal weight. When you are attuned with your body, your intuition will guide you to eat exactly what you need and as many calories as you need. For those who are inclined to count calories, caloric information is provided for the recipes, along with per serving measures of fats, carbohydrates, dietary fiber, and protein.

## Why Processed and Genetically Modified (GMO) Foods Are So Bad for Us

**PROCESSING** is a term that is typically used to describe the act of taking an ingredient through an established (usually routine) set of procedures that converts that ingredient from one form to another. Industrially processed foods have been altered from their original form and now have a different molecular structure than the form of the food that nature provided. The food is different than in its natural state.

Processed foods have little to no nutritional value at all because they undergo a

# 25 Reasons to Love the Earth Diet

1. It is simple to understand.

2. The guidelines are easy to follow.

3. The recipes are delicious.

4. It's appropriate for those who choose to eat exclusively raw or vegan—and also for those who want to eat some meat, fish, and eggs along with their plant-based foods.

5. You can eat how much you want, whenever you want—as long as you adhere to the principles of the Earth Diet.

6. You can eat dessert every day if you want to—and not gain weight. The Earth Diet allows you to be decadent, as well as healthy!

7. Your body will naturally return to its optimal weight without struggle.

8. You'll feel energized because your body is being highly nourished.

9. You'll look terrific, with healthy hair and radiant skin.

10. Your brain will function at its peak.

11. Your vision can improve.

12. You'll sleep like a baby.

13. Your aches and pains from inflammation can disappear.

14. You won't be held back anymore by fatigue.

15. Your mood will be uplifted.

16. You may never get another head cold.

17. You'll feel more confident and empowered when you see how much is possible.

18. Because you're listening to your body, you'll come to trust your innate wisdom.

19. You'll feel excited to eat your meals—instead of afraid.

20. Guilt is not on the menu! You'll stop beating yourself up for eating certain foods, because adding shame and criticism to a less healthy choice is counter to the tenets of the Earth Diet. If you do eat junk food from time to time, you're permitted to enjoy it.

21. You'll be encouraged to think more positive thoughts than negative ones.

22. Because you're using locally grown produce, you'll be reducing your carbon footprint and contributing to the sustainability of the environment.

23. Because you're eating local foods, you'll be supporting the economy in your region.

24. Because you're eating seasonal produce, you'll experience diverse flavors throughout the year.

25. You will feel at one with Mother Earth—part of nature.

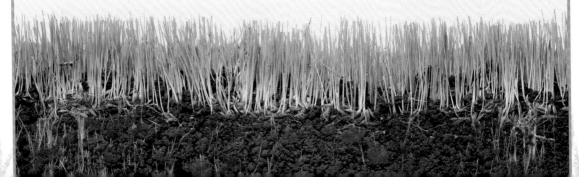

complicated procedure to arrive at our tables, from how they are grown to how they are packaged, which consists of:

- Growing the produce (with pesticides and hormones), and then harvesting it.
- Shipping the produce to the manufacturers, which may entail international flying—and if that is the case, exposure to high radiation.
- Reshaping and restructuring.
- Adding other ingredients, like flavorings, preservatives, and stabilizers.
- Packaging in toxic plastic.
- Distribution, which requires more handling and travel.
- Sitting on store shelves where we purchase it.

Most processed foods contain ingredients that I believe are toxic to the human body. As a result, there is little to no nutritional benefit in eating processed food—anything good you might otherwise get from them is counteracted by their negative properties. Processed ingredients include refined sugar; non-organic dairy; GMO ingredients like corn and soy; and ingredients that are hard to pronounce, such as additives, flavorings, preservatives, anti-caking agents, fillers, and colorings.

We innately know it is wrong to eat processed foods since they leave us feeling unfulfilled. When they enter the digestive system, they send a message to the brain saying, "No nutrition received, send more." That's why we usually can eat so much processed food in one sitting.

There are hundreds of reasons why processed food is not good for the human body. Here's just a partial list of conditions they can contribute to:

- Weak immune system
- Weight gain
- Headaches and migraines
- Acne, psoriasis, and other skin issues
- Diseases
- Cancer
- Stress and anxiety
- Fatigue (the body must use a lot of energy to digest them)
- Aging
- Addiction and dependency on processed foods, and cravings for more
- Yeast overgrowth, candida
- Digestion issues like IBS and bloating
- Food sensitivities and allergies
- Cellulite
- Diabetes

Over 70 percent of processed foods now contain ingredients that can be classified as **GENETICALLY MODIFIED ORGANISMS** (GMOs). GMO foods are created through the manipulation of plant and animal development by altering their gene expression. In my opinion, a food that has been genetically modified is nutritionally suspect and likely to be toxic and harmful to the body. Human interference with food in its natural state turns it into something else that may not be healthy to eat. For instance, genetic engineering can introduce an allergen into a food that previously did not contain it. Do some research to see if consuming GMOs feels right to you.

When I lecture and do cooking demonstrations, I'm often asked to back up my opinions on why people should avoid GMO foods in their diet. To me it is just common sense, but I've also read numerous articles and books over the years that have reinforced this opinion. One of the most powerful was published in May 2013 on *The Food Revolution Network* blog created by John Robbins, author of the now-classic groundbreaking book *Diet for a New America* (1987), and his son, Ocean Robbins, who has a similar mission to protect the food supply. The article was written by Thierry Vrain, Ph.D., who formerly worked for a big agribusiness company in Canada and now is attempting to expose the hazards of GMOs. Vrain writes:

> *In 2009 the American Academy of Environmental Medicine called for a moratorium of GM foods, safety testing, and labeling. Their review of the available literature at the time noted that animals show serious health risks associated with GM food consumption including infertility, immune dysregulation, accelerated aging, dysregulation of genes associated with cholesterol synthesis, insulin regulation, cell signaling, and protein formation, and changes in the liver, kidney, spleen, and gastrointestinal system.*[2]

That's incredibly scary, right? Why take a chance on it? Making the commitment to eat unprocessed, organic foods is a guarantee that you won't have to worry about chemicals or weird genetic issues when you're having a meal or a snack.

## Please, Personalize the Earth Diet

I purposefully created the Earth Diet in such a way that it can fit into everyone's lifestyle. So follow the guidelines to whatever extent makes you happy and comfortable. Make your decisions according to your values, your preferences, and your biological needs. This is very important: *You should always listen to your body and trust your intuition. Do what feels right and best for you.*

It can be tempting to judge or comment upon other people's eating habits, or even to beat yourself up for your own. If you catch yourself being critical, remember how yoga teachers tell you to keep your eyes on your own mat and concentrate on your own practice and where you are, rather than focusing on comparisons with others. Remember, it's just as renowned self-development author and speaker Wayne Dyer so wisely says, "When you judge another, you do not define them. You define yourself."[3] Some people thrive from *not* having meat, for instance, while others enjoy it. Many people find that the longer they stay on the Earth Diet, the less meat they want to eat. If you do choose to eat meat, make sure it is organic and free range. If your meat is not organic, then it is likely to contain hormones, toxic chemicals, and antibiotics, as well as genetically modified organisms. This meat is not good for us.

Similarly, if you personally feel good about eating eggs then you are free to eat them, as long as you remember that they will only be as good as the birds they come from. Healthy birds produce healthy eggs. But just like the rule with eating meat, it is best to avoid eggs laid by chickens raised with hormones and antibiotics or fed

GMO grains. Organic eggs from free-range chickens can provide many nutrients.

Remember, the Earth Diet always gives a range of healthy options. Depending on where you live, the concepts of *local* and *seasonal* could greatly impact your choices. Imagine you lived in the Antarctic: Fish would probably be a daily staple of your diet, and there would be fewer fruits and vegetables available to you than someone who lives in Manhattan near a Whole Foods Market. In North Queensland, where I spent some of my early years, there was a tremendous amount of fresh produce because of the tropical climate, so the concept of *local* meant eating mangoes, avocados, bananas, and coconuts. Yum.

One of the most wonderful things people often tell me is how they can't believe they get to enjoy their favorite flavors and tastes with the Earth Diet recipes, while still providing their bodies with all the essentials of proper nutrition. They can't believe how many choices are available. My response is that we are fortunate, indeed, to be living in a day and age where we can have our cake and eat it, too! The Earth Diet includes many delicious dessert recipes, and I've even created a seven-day guide for dessert lovers.

In his book *The Slow Down Diet*, Marc David, M.D., explains the neurobiological reasons pleasure and digestion are linked. For one, just eating increases our endorphin levels—those are the same "happy chemicals" that give runners a feeling of elation. As David points out, "The same chemical that makes you feel good burns body fat. Furthermore, the greater the endorphin release in your digestive tract, the more blood and oxygen will be delivered there. This means increased digestion, assimilation, and ultimately greater efficiency

in calorie burning."[4] He also points out that the body's stress response (the opposite of the relaxation response) "desensitizes us to pleasure."[5] If we feel less satisfied by eating our food, this causes us to seek more food to create greater fulfillment.

You'd be surprised by the questions I hear. Many people have asked me if they can drink alcohol on the Earth Diet. I advise them to make the best choice they can from the options that are available. If you do want to imbibe alcohol, choose the healthiest, least processed kinds, such as organic wines (fermented grapes) or homebrewed organic beer, vodka, and tequila. Avoid alcoholic beverages that incorporate soda or sweet syrup. Are you starting to get a sense of what I mean by making choices that are right for you?

I used to waste a lot of time feeling unhealthy and toxic. Now I prefer to feel as alive as possible. In my opinion, being truly alive means inhabiting a body built on cells that are well nourished with vital nutrients. What we put into our bodies is what we become, as our cells are made up of the atoms from the things we eat. Every human being benefits from eating foods full of vitamins, minerals, and other nutrients. It should make sense to everyone that fueling the body with proper nutrition through whole, organic foods is our best choice for optimum health. Being truly alive means also enjoying what we eat, and being happy. It means listening to our bodies and trusting our innate wisdom.

By eating the best natural foods on the planet, I know that my body is being taken care of, and I can get on with living in every other dimension of human life.

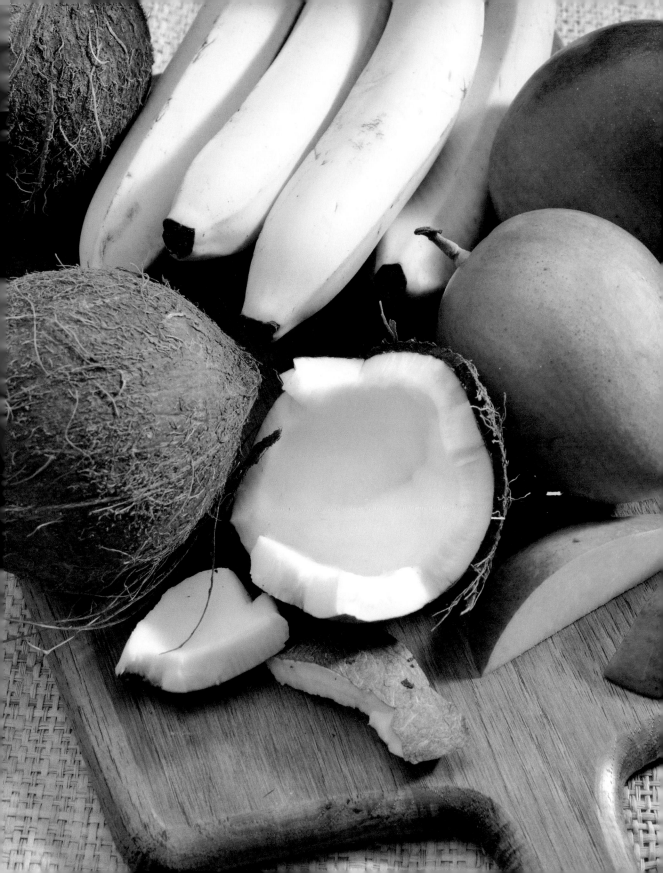

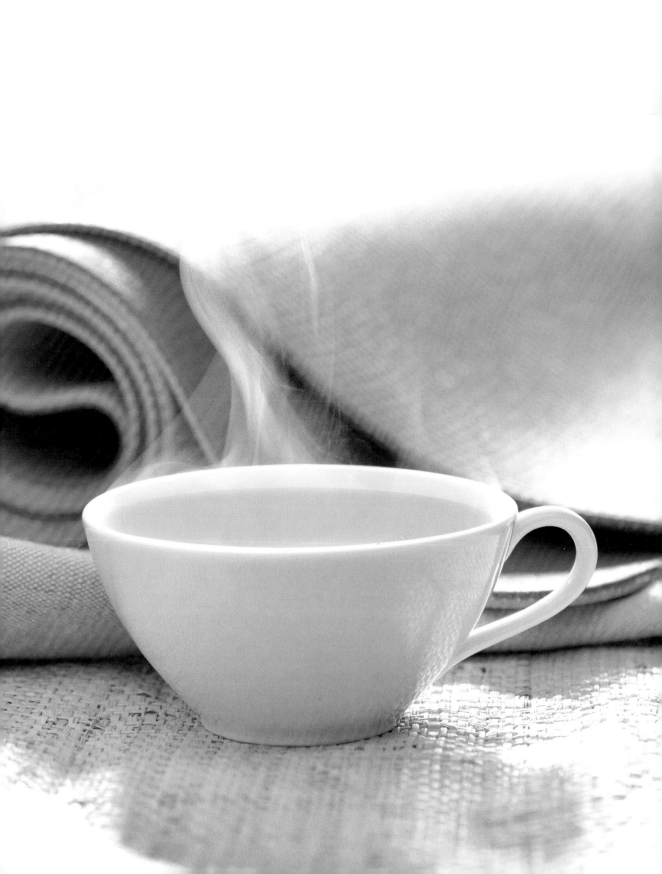

# CHAPTER 2

# Self-Healing with the Earth Diet

**"Loving ourselves works miracles in our lives."**

—Louise Hay

As you know, I learned at age 21 that I had a precancerous tumor in my throat the size of a golf ball. On top of that, I had cellulite on my stomach and legs, mononucleosis (also known as Epstein-Barr virus, or in Australia, glandular fever), a digestive system that was not working (constipation), and the early stages of chronic fatigue syndrome. I was addicted to junk food and trapped in a vicious cycle of almost daily binge eating. Because I'd been eating genetically modified and processed foods, I was extremely bloated, stressed, depressed, disempowered, tired, and sore.

When I realized I'd hit rock bottom with my health, I decided I wouldn't live another day like that and chose to make a change. Right away I committed to self-heal using the earth's natural means. I began juicing every day and developed new recipes for a variety of raw and cooked dishes made from fresh, organic ingredients. I also adopted a positive mental outlook and consciously started thinking better thoughts. In addition, I did natural treatments and switched over all my skin care and house-hold cleaners to natural, plant-based products. Once I made my decision to self-heal, within three months I was completely cured of all the adverse conditions I was experiencing. I'm pleased to report to you that to this day, seven years later, I've maintained my new lifestyle and I am extremely healthy.

Basically, I live the most natural and organic lifestyle possible, which is the Earth Diet. By *natural*, I mean consuming products and foods that are untouched and in their original state. By *organic*, I am referring to the regulations set forth by the National Organic Program of the U.S. Department of Agriculture.[1] I have helped thousands of people to tap into their own self-healing abilities and wisdom, too.

It does not take an advanced degree to understand that whole, natural, organic foods are better for us than processed junk foods filled with synthetic chemicals, hormones, and genetic modifications. I believe everything you need to know to feel better, even if that means partial relief of your symptoms, is built into your body. The healing process is different for every person, and you know your body better than anyone else does or could. The more you can do to support your own innate healing mechanisms, the better.

# Conditions that Have Been Helped with the Earth Diet

Here is a selected list of common health conditions that people have told me have improved for them, or even been entirely reversed, by using the Earth Diet recipes and self-healing protocols. A full list is provided on my website: TheEarthDiet.com/BookGift.

Accelerated aging

Acid reflux

Aches and pains

Acne

Addiction

Allergies

Alzheimer's disease

Anger

Anorexia

Anxiety

Arterial plaque

Arthritis

Asthma

Attention deficit hyperactivity disorder (ADHD)

Autism

Autoimmune disease

Benign tumors

Binge eating

Blackheads

Bleeding gums

Bloating

Blood clots

Bulimia

Body odor

Bone disorders

Cancer

Candida

Cardiovascular cholesterol

Celiac disease

Cerebral palsy

Chronic fatigue

Colds

Cold sores

Constipation

Crohn's disease

Cysts

Dandruff

Depression

Diabetes

Diarrhea

Eczema

Emotional eating

Fatty tumors

Fear

Fibroid tumors

Fibromyalgia

Fingernails (brittle or soft)

Flu

Fluid retention

Gallstones

Gas

Gluten intolerance

Gout

Gray hair

Guilt

Gum disorders

Hair loss

Headaches

Heartburn

Heart disease

Heart palpitations

Herpes

High blood pressure

High cholesterol

Hormonal imbalance

Hyperactivity

Hypertension

Hypoglycemia

Impotence

Infections

Infertility

Inflammation

Insomnia

Irregular heartbeats

Irritable bowel syndrome

Irritation

Kidney stones

Loss of smell

Low blood sugar

Low energy

Malignant tumors

Menstrual cramps

Metabolism issues

Migraines

Mood swings

Multiple sclerosis

Muscle cramps

Muscular disorders

Nervousness

Obesity

Osteoporosis

Overeating

Overweight

Panic attacks

Parkinson's disease

Poor circulation

Premenstrual syndrome (PMS)

Psoriasis

Sexually transmitted diseases

Sluggish gallbladder

Spasms

Stiffness

Stress

Stuttering

Teeth grinding

Tension

Thrush

Thyroid issues

Tightness

Tuberculosis

Tumors

Ulcers

Varicose veins

Viruses

Warts

Wrinkled skin

Yeast infections

## What Exactly Is Self-Healing?

Self-healing is a phrase that refers to the body's natural process of recovery. In the context of this book, it means that the methods used to promote physical healing were tailored to the unique experience and requirements of the individual by the individual. Self-healing may be achieved through mechanisms such as eating organic foods, indulging in natural treatments and therapies (baths, massages, and acupuncture, for example), relaxation, meditation, prayer, love, self-empowerment, self-motivation, and positive thinking. We are very intelligent and wise beings by nature, so please use your intuition and trust your body to let you know which of these techniques is going to be most beneficial for you.

More people every day are realizing that there's more to getting well than what pharmaceutical drugs alone can do for us. There is a growing body of research that shows how debilitating stress can be over time—and you should be aware that stress factors include forces both outside us, like pollution, and inside us, like our habitual thoughts.

Our attitudes and emotions play a big role in healing. If you feel as if you have no control over your destiny and health, you may spiral downward emotionally and feel increased stress. If you take even a few positive actions on your own behalf, you'll feel empowered and feel reduced stress. This can be an emotionally uplifting experience that raises the level of your wellness significantly. In one way or another, or better yet, in many ways, each of us can contribute something to the healing of our body.

Your body is indicating that it needs healing if, among other things, you experience any of the following:

- You feel tired and weak.
- You have physical pain or inflammation.
- You get frequent colds or headaches.
- You are bloated.
- You have acid reflux or heartburn.
- You are constipated.
- You have cancer or another chronic disease.
- You have a virus or infection.
- You have a yeast overgrowth.
- You have acne, eczema, psoriasis, or dandruff.
- You have dark circles under your eyes.
- You are losing your hair.
- Your eyesight or hearing is weak.
- You are carrying excess weight.
- You feel bad (stuck, disempowered, or depressed) the majority of the time.
- You have a substance addiction or a process addiction.

To self-heal using proper nutrition, search for recipes that you particularly love or that excite you in Part II of this book. Good thoughts and good food are good medicine. Follow the guide for Boosting Your Immunity to heal and improve any health condition (see p. 184).

Remember always to consult with your doctor before stopping any form of ongoing treatment. Do not disregard professional medical advice. If you are currently taking medication, for instance, continue until you know for sure that you are better off without it. Coming off a medication or reducing the level of medication being taken for a variety of conditions is a process many people have been able to go through once they began following the Earth Diet, but it is best handled carefully and gradually. When you feel confident in your body's ability to heal and you've been feeding your cells optimal nourishment for a period of time, then you may be in a good place physically to become entirely free of medication.

Personally, I have not taken medication from a pharmacy for over nine years. Since I began using the Earth Diet, food has been my only medicine. This has worked well for me.

Remember that every person is different and therefore everybody's healing journey is different. But supplying your body with proper nutrition is a foundational step no matter who you are or what your health concerns are. Nutritional biochemist T. Colin Campbell, Ph.D., author of *The China Study* and its sequel, *Whole,* has conducted research that demonstrates how rates of Alzheimer's disease, strokes, osteoporosis, and other diseases are radically lower in places where the population eats a largely plant-based diet and no refined foods.[2] It seems that many diseases can be improved, if not entirely reversed, with proper nutrition, including adult-onset diabetes, heart disease, and some forms of cancer, since, as Campbell writes, "A good diet is the most powerful weapon we have against disease and sickness."[3]

## The Perfect Recipe for Self-healing

The perfect recipe for self-healing is to properly nourish the body, the mind, and the spirit every day. Use the following suggestions as a protocol for designing a personalized self-healing program. Stay flexible and approach your healing process as an experiment in living.

**EAT THE EARTH DIET RECIPES.** Give your body high doses of nourishment regularly. After eating a single recipe you will feel good! Every recipe provides the body with essential nutrients and uses the cleanest ingredients possible. If you live the Earth Diet

100 percent—meaning that everything you put into and on your body is in the most natural state possible—you can begin to transform your health in as little as one week. The juice recipes are the most powerful ones for feeling good immediately. As Jack Kornfield so wisely says in *Buddha's Little Instruction Book:* "No matter how difficult the past, you can always begin again today."[4] The better you eat now, the better you will feel about yourself today.

**PRACTICE THINKING GOOD THOUGHTS.** By replacing negative thoughts with better-feeling thoughts, you train your mind to be more positive overall. Eventually you will be made up of positivity. The human body is composed of over 50 trillion cells. Each is bathed in the blood chemistry of the thoughts you are thinking and the emotions you are feeling. If you are scared, for instance, your cells are bathed in adrenaline. If you are in love, they are bathed in oxytocin. It is therefore important during self-healing to choose to think positive thoughts that lead to positive feelings. Your cells will physically reflect what you are feeding them mentally and emotionally.

It has been proven that negative thoughts can harm us. If you persistently think negative thoughts and expect the worst, this affects your body. Negativity does not feel good. A positive thought will move you to healing and to living in the body you want. We'll talk more about this in the next chapter.

**COMMIT TO MAKING CHANGE ONE SMALL STEP AT A TIME.** Remember, wherever you are in your life is perfect, because you are learning. Even if you feel you made a misstep, you can always start fresh right now. You always have a choice about what to do next in response to whatever is happening to you. Let go of guilt that will only keep you trapped in the past.

**BELIEVE YOU CAN DO IT WITH EVERY CELL OF YOUR BODY**. You really can do anything you set your mind to. The quality of your beliefs is important because the mind is so powerful. You have probably heard of the placebo effect, which is the belief that something will work to heal you. Studies have proven that when we have confidence that something is good for us, it can benefit us. In scientific experiments, researchers test active chemical ingredients against inactive ones to control for the *placebo effect*. In many cases, even when patients were tested with an inactive sugar pill, their symptoms were healed. That's how powerful the mind is. As Norman Cousins, a man who experienced a dramatic spontaneous healing, explains in his 1979 book *The Anatomy of an Illness*: "The process works not because of any magic in the tablet but because the human body is its own best apothecary and because the most successful prescriptions are filled by the body itself."[5]

In *The Biology of Belief*, cell biologist Bruce H. Lipton, Ph.D., explains the mechanisms through which our thoughts affect the cells in our bodies and why our beliefs about health matter as much as, if not more than, conventional medicine. He writes: "Because we are not powerless biochemical machines, popping a pill every time we are mentally or physically out of tune is not the answer. Drugs and surgery are powerful tools when they are not overused, but the notion of simple drug fixes is fundamentally flawed. Every time a drug is introduced into the body to correct function A, it inevitably throws off functions B, C, or D. It is not gene-directed hormones and neurotransmitters that control our bodies and our minds; our beliefs control our bodies, our minds, and thus our lives. . . ."[6] To self-heal, we need to eat nourishing food and feed our minds nourishing thoughts.

**DO NOT ACCEPT STRESS IN YOUR LIFE.** Over a period of time, stress depletes us and can develop into autoimmune dysfunctions, adrenal burnout, chronic pain, and diseases of the heart—even cancer. Stress can kill if it is left unchecked. If you are faced with a life-threatening disease, it is even more important than at other times that you remain in a state of ease and relaxation. If you have reached the point where your life is already being threatened by an illness, it is crucial you make transforming choices to sustain your health. You have no time to waste.

**REMEMBER THAT YOU ARE IMPORTANT.** You are part of the community of the Earth and we need you. Some people feel disempowered with their existence and fear that their lives do not matter. But each of us has a gift, something good to offer humanity and the planet.

**TRUST YOURSELF AND DO YOUR BEST TO LOVE YOURSELF FROM THE INSIDE OUT.** Love is an important component of self-healing. Be in a state of love whenever possible, as love supports healing by restoring and rejuvenating the immune system. Fear interrupts growth mechanisms and weakens the immune system. Stress promotes unhealthy chemistry in the body.

**APPRECIATE YOUR BODY.** If you really knew what your body was doing 24 hours a day to keep you alive, you would want to hug yourself and consume only nourishing fuel! Be grateful for the body you do have, and for what *is* working right now. Count your blessings. Are you grateful that you can walk? Are you grateful that you woke up breathing without the help of a machine? Be grateful for your lungs, your toes, your ears, your eyes, your stomach . . . the list goes on.

# Universal Healing Strategies

Because they weaken the immune system and can cause all types of illnesses, in my opinion, everyone should avoid:

- Eating excess processed foods with refined sugars, refined flours, refined grains, additives, MSG, aspartame, preservatives, chemicals, and pesticides

- Fast food

- Malnutrition

- Drinking and eating non-organic dairy

- Being more acidic than alkaline

- Obesity and excess weight

- Cooking with Teflon

- Not spending time surrounded by nature

- Sodium nitrite found in most processed foods

- Food colorings

- Watching television for excessive amounts of time

- Lack of exercise

- Sitting for prolonged amounts of time

- Hydrogenated oils and trans fatty acids

- Plastic food containers, including lining inside of cans (acrylamides)

- Home cleaning products with toxic chemical ingredients, including laundry detergents, dryer sheets, dry cleaning chemicals

- Cosmetics and personal care products that contain aluminum and synthetic ingredients

- Smoking cigarettes

- Perfumes and fragrances

- Excess chlorine exposure

- Thinking negative thoughts, being unconscious, stress, self-doubt, doubt, regret, guilt, blame, not being at peace with self, not accepting this present moment

In my opinion we should all do the following things because it appears that they can help prevent cancer, diabetes, heart disease, and obesity, and keep the immune system consistently strong:

- Juice daily

- Eat organic foods

- Eat superfoods

- Eat anti-inflammatory foods

- Eat anti-cancer foods

- Get more vitamin D and sunshine

- Be in nature

- Eat green vegetables

- Drink green tea

- Keep the digestive system healthy

- Be more alkaline than acidic

- Eat medicinal mushrooms, like reishi and shiitake

- Drink bentonite clay

- Eat pomegranate seeds

- Drink chlorella

- Eat foods containing omega-3 oils, like chia seeds

- Consume lycopene and tomatoes

- Drink diatomaceous earth

- Relax and rest

- Meditate/pray

- Exercise, do yoga, do tai chi

- Take healing baths

- Sweat in saunas

- Be at ease, practicing presence and stillness

- Laugh and embrace joy, love, self-love, positive thoughts, affirmations, and following our bliss

## Managing Detox Symptoms

When we start eating healthy, and especially juicing, it's common to experience mild detox symptoms. The shift in our diet can leave us feeling unwell, drunk, agitated, and itchy. Manage this by facilitating the body in getting toxins out and nutrition in. Juicing helps. Gentle exercise during the first few days or weeks of making a change is beneficial. Walking is highly recommended especially in nature, like at the park or on the beach. Sleeping, relaxation, and getting a massage help. Drinking bentonite clay to absorb toxins is helpful, too. Watch funny movies to keep you focused on happiness. Healing foods that are extremely soothing during a detox are potatoes, quinoa, rice, and cacao (chocolate).

If you are someone with a serious health condition, someone who wants to break an addiction or a destructive habit, or a pharmaceutical user, you may expect resistance of this type from both your body and your mind when you begin shifting your diet and lifestyle. Stick with your plan. The types of detox symptoms you may experience will subside as soon as your body is less toxic. Your body and mind both will adjust. The more confident you become in your own ability to heal, the more deliberately you'll be able to choose how you think and feel. Also the healthier you become, the happier you will be and the easier life will seem. Although there may be an element of you that is challenged by the prospect of letting go and living a new, healthier life, you can trust that this detox period will pass.

*Caution:* If you are taking prescription drugs, seek assistance from a qualified health-care professional to guide you in tapering off them in an appropriate manner that does not

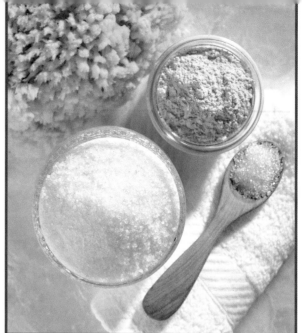

cause you undue discomfort or put you in any kind of danger. You don't want to create new health problems for yourself while you are consciously engaged in making health improvements.

What also helps to manage detox symptoms is sweating in a sauna or steam room, or in a warm/hot bath. Taking baths is very beneficial. Here are a few recipes for bathing.

**DETOX BATH:** Fill your bathtub with hot water, as hot as you can handle without being scalded. Add 2 cups of Epsom salts. Soak in the bath for at least 10 minutes. This will help flush out toxins.

**RELAXATION BATH:** Fill your bathtub with warm to hot water. Add 1 cup salt and 1 cup fresh lavender flowers (or 1 teaspoon of lavender essential oil). Stay in the bath for 25 minutes. Practice affirmations and positive thinking while you soak.

**CLEAR SKIN BATH:** Fill your bathtub with warm to hot water. Add 1 cup bentonite clay and stir around until the entire bath is cloudy. Soak for 30 minutes.

## Every Day Is a New Opportunity to Heal

We all have a choice every day about what we put into our body. We can decide, *Today I will have a juice, smoothie, tea, and raw meal*—or not. We have the option to eat healthy foods. Consider we also choose to feel good or not. A healthy life is a choice from moment to moment.

Luckily for us, there are billions of moments each day, and each is an opportunity to make a new choice. We get to keep re-choosing. This is how many thousands have ended food addictions and bad habits, by realizing if we eat something unhealthy, the next choice we can make is to eat something healthy. We are not trapped in a vicious cycle; we have the power to choose.

If you don't believe you have control over choices, put your arms above your head right now and stretch them high while taking in a deep breath. Then breathe out. That conscious action represents you driving the wheel in your own life.

Some people have an extremely hard time getting started. It does get easier, and the healthier you get, the easier it gets. The healthier you get, the better you feel. The better you feel, the healthier you get. When we feel good, we are more attracted to foods that keep us feeling good. Some people get frustrated and want to give up. They fear they won't be able to live a life that doesn't include junk food. Wayne Dyer advises us to "hit the delete button every time fear appears."[7]

When you observe yourself thinking, *I can't do it,* interrupt the thought and substitute a better one. It has to be something you believe is honest, and also supportive of your goals. Perhaps you would be inspired by thinking, *I am doing the best I can* or *I am capable of eating healthy today.*

Consider that we're not stuck in any of these conditions:

- Being tired the majority of the time
- Feeling sick the majority of the time
- Feeling depressed the majority of the time
- Feeling bad the majority of the time
- Feeling guilty the majority of the time

Also consider this:

- We all want to feel good. When we get sick, our bodies' natural reaction is to do things to get better. It is our natural state to feel good. It is in our best interest to feel good.
- Stress is more likely to come from lifestyle choices than from our genes.
- You can choose to live the Earth Diet lifestyle fully or just incorporate bits of it into your life. Either way you are going to feel better.

Many people say that prior to using the Earth Diet they just accepted that they felt bad and sick the majority of the time and did nothing about it. Using these recipes and experiencing the health and energy that come from them, however, they learned how good the human body was designed to feel. You can feel that well also. This is an opportunity for you to begin a powerful journey to optimal health.

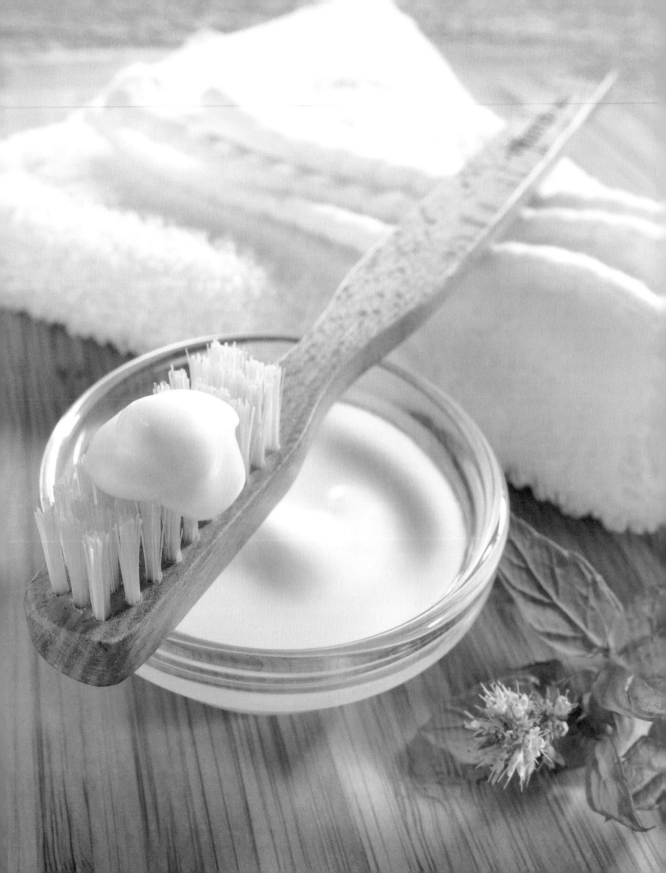

# CHAPTER 3

# The Earth Diet Lifestyle

## Heaven on Earth starts within you.

The Earth Diet lifestyle encompasses all the choices we live by day to day, not only what we eat, but what we put on our bodies, the products we use, the clothes we wear, the type of house we live in, the cars we drive, and more. Our lifestyle encompasses everything we do.

During the first 365 days after I started the Earth Diet blog, I not only changed my eating habits, I also changed everything I put on my skin and used in my home. What is the point of healthy eating if we keep putting chemicals on our skin? It is the same thing! We are what we eat and what we absorb!

As a general rule, always remember: If you cannot eat it, do not put it on your skin. If you cannot eat it, do not spray it in your house. Why? Because the skin absorbs everything it touches. It is our largest organ. Our lungs are also absorbing tiny molecules that we breathe in. Whatever we put on our bodies or use around our home, we are basically "eating" through our lungs and skin.

In this chapter you'll find recipes to make your own natural skin care and household cleaning products. There are many more recipes than it's possible to include in this book, so if you are looking for something in particular that's not here, visit TheEarthDiet.com.

Most people want to be healthy because they know they will feel better. This desire is at the core of everything I've learned since helping thousands of people to heal. Everyone wants to feel better. Where do we begin? By looking at our lives and identifying the areas and choices that can be improved. There may be healthier options for literally everything we do. So each of us must choose what to focus on and then transition to a healthier lifestyle one step, one choice, one natural alternative at a time.

We can look at many aspects of our lifestyle. Obviously, one major aspect I looked at when I began making changes was food. I transformed that and am still enjoying the results of the shift. I then started slowly but surely to sift chemicals out of my life by replacing synthetic products with organic ones. For example, I stopped wearing conventional deodorant. Today I use organic deodorant or wipe my underarms with a slice of lemon. Some days I even use none. I stopped using conventional deodorant because I learned how it can clog the lymphatic system and sweat glands with aluminum and other heavy metals. Nature made our armpits to release sweat and toxins, and it's unhealthy to interfere. My armpits actually used to ache when I wore conventional deodorant.

Another example of a change I made is that when I want to wear makeup now, I do not use conventional makeup because of all the chemicals manufacturers put it in. I have found cosmetics made from plant-based ingredients that do a better job at "making me up," plus they nourish my skin instead of aging it.

I like to wear moisturizer, but I do not use conventional body lotion. I use coconut oil, avocado oil, olive oil, or cacao butter. I switch it up between these four oils to allow my skin to absorb a variety of different nutrients. I value my skin, and I want to nourish it the best I can. When you make your own moisturizer, you can scent it with essential oils, such as peppermint, lavender, and lemon.

In this chapter, we'll look individually at different choices and break them down so you can see how you can begin to adopt the Earth Diet lifestyle.

## Choosing the Lifestyle That's Right for You

Your lifestyle choices may be different from someone else's for good reasons. For example, someone with cancer might choose different aspects of their life to improve as compared to someone with acne. I have worked with people who wanted to address both of these issues, and others. If I work with someone who has cancer, we take all chemicals and junk foods out of their diets immediately. They begin juicing on a daily basis to ensure they're getting plenty of nourishment throughout the day.

After that, we look at other lifestyle factors, like skin-care products. Because the skin is the largest organ in the human body, we consume a lot of chemicals through it. People with cancer usually choose to switch their lifestyle to be 100 percent organic in order to heal quicker. Since they may be receiving toxic treatments, such as radiation and chemotherapy, they want to ensure they are reducing their exposure to poison everywhere else, in addition to eating nutrient-dense foods that boost their energy and immunity.

In the case of acne, people have a little more wiggle room since the health challenge is less severe. They may want to keep eating their favorite cookie made by their favorite bakery from time to time, so that remains in their lifestyle. If so, I suggest they balance out the sweet treat by drinking a beet juice or a green juice once a day to ensure receiving the nutrients they need for their acne to heal.

For someone whose acne covers his or her face entirely, if the skin is aching and embarrassing, and this person wants to heal the condition as soon as possible, then we would look in more detail at their lifestyle choices, including removing sugar entirely—no cookies—and I'd advise doing a 30-day program consisting of twice daily juicing, along with drinking one smoothie and eating a majority of raw plant-based recipes; a liver cleanse; and a series of recipes for applying nutrients to the skin, like an avocado mask. By changing their lifestyle, people with severe acne can expect to experience improvements within a few weeks and significant results in four to six months.

After healing from one condition, many of my clients choose to tackle new goals by making additional lifestyle modifications, such as exercising more, making their own shampoo, and eating to get rid of their cellulite.

Our lifestyle choices affect what we look like and how we feel.

## Buying the Egg vs. Making the Egg

Since I began living the Earth Diet lifestyle, I've cooked more of my own meals and eat out rarely. I do this for many reasons, including that I like to know what's going into my food and I actually enjoy it. It is especially fun to create decadent plant-based desserts!

Let's say we have a choice between going out to a café and purchasing cooked eggs, or making them at home from eggs laid by our own chickens. At the café, the cook is using eggs flown in from another state; cooks them in GMO vegetable oil (this is the worst-case scenario), which makes them instantly toxic; and then garnishes them with table salt and serves them with some home fries that were deep fried in vegetable oil and a non-organic salad whose ingredients were sprayed with a dozen chemicals, like pesticides, when they were grown. After our eggs have undergone that process, we don't get much nutritional value from them. We may even be left feeling kind of tired as our body digests the food.

Compare this to preparing the meal at home using eggs you've gathered from your very own hens. Let's say the chickens were fed scraps of the organic vegetables you ate, which you raised in your own garden. They are also allowed to range freely in their pen and eat their natural diet of worms and insects. Imagine your well-fed chickens produce seven eggs a day—enough for your entire family—and you cook these in extra-virgin coconut oil before seasoning them with Himalayan salt and fresh cilantro from your garden.

Which eggs do you think you would enjoy most?

The problem with choosing to eat at a conventional café or diner is that our purchases are supporting their unsustainable and unhealthy behavior. If we want to live in a more organic world, our choices need to reflect it. There is always more value in choosing the healthier option.

Just do the best you can and keep taking more steps to choose a healthier lifestyle. I currently do not own chickens, because I live in a city, so I cannot use my own eggs. My choice is therefore either to go out to an organic café and have them make me some eggs or, even better, to buy organic eggs from the health-food store and cook them myself. Making my own food definitely seems worth the time and effort.

The truth is that I created the Earth Diet to suit my current life. I travel the world and often live in apartments and hotels where growing my own garden or raising my own chickens is not possible—although it is a goal for the future. I live the best I can, given my current situation. There are always ways to upgrade a lifestyle, and I am aware of where those areas exist for me. I am also open to the evolution of better, more practical ideas about treating my body and the Earth.

I am careful about all my purchasing decisions. I want to wear fashionable clothing and be proud of what I have on, but I do not want a child slave to make my clothes or to wear the skin of an animal that was tortured. I love wearing clothing made from bamboo or hemp—or something my mum made from recycled materials!

Whatever I buy, I always prefer to find the healthiest, most humanely produced version possible. But we can't be too uptight about our lives. We must live in flow, like organic plants, which aren't straight and rigid, but bend with the wind! I want to use technology like iPhones and laptops, and when I buy a house someday I intend to install solar panels and a water filtration system in it. I want to go out and eat and drink with friends, as this is fun, but I prefer to go to organic restaurants that serve decadent and good-tasting, as well as healthy, dishes.

It can be overwhelming to look at all the possible changes we could make. In a perfect world, I would snap my fingers and then I would be living in my dream eco-house, driving a Tesla electric car that was charged by the sun, and making all of my own meals from ingredients grown in my own garden. But that is not my reality. I don't have time to make all of my own food for every meal at the present moment. I have to take my life one choice at a time and do the best I can.

## Positive Thinking

Removing chemicals and toxic foods can help us to remove negative thoughts. Many people feel guilty about feeling depressed, but that just makes it worse! How can we feel good if we are surrounded by a toxic environment and junk foods? These chemicals inhibit the brain from functioning properly. It may not be entirely your fault that you feel depressed, have an illness, or are overweight. You probably aren't aware of the amount of chemicals that you are absorbing on a daily basis.

The Earth Diet lifestyle is about living a well-rounded healthy lifestyle. Imagine that you are eating natural organic foods, you live in your dream eco-home, your relationships are rich, your schedule is great—meaning, you control what you do each day and take time to relax and enjoy yourself and your life—you love your work, your career is fulfilling, and you always get your work done in a timely manner and feel like you are making a difference in the world. In fact, you feel good about everything.

Sure, there are areas that you want to improve, perhaps you want to lose a pound or two, but you are thinking about doing so in a relaxed and cheerful manner. You accept that you have to do one step at a time, rather than being overwhelmed and wanting everything to just be done. That's *positive thinking*.

One thing I've had to realize is that my life is happening now. This is it! I've learned that negative thoughts do not serve me and do not get me anywhere other than cause me to experience pain.

Being healthy doesn't just mean eating healthy food; it also means having positive thoughts in your head. It can take a little practice to train yourself not to indulge in negativity, because it really can become a habit. But it's worth it. Negative thinking has been linked to all kinds of diseases, including cancer and back pain, and it is just not the mental place we want to dwell in. In his book *Spontaneous Healing*, Andrew Weil, M.D., comments, "The mind can depress the immune system and can unbalance the autonomic nervous system, leading to disturbances in digestion, circulation, and all other internal functions. You must know how to use the mind in service of healing."[1] If you are depressed or angry or anxious, it can be a hard road to recovery. I can understand that. All I am suggesting is that you make an effort to look at your thoughts to see if they are constructive to your well-being.

When we think negative thoughts we feel

bad and our body chemistry changes. When we feel bad, our immune system becomes suppressed.

Many people believe that positive thinking is a choice. If the choice does lie within us, then for the sake of our health we should choose positivity. Of course, expect this to be a lifelong process. It's not like you can wave a magic wand and—*Shazzam*—be "cured" and never think a negative thought again. I wish it could be like that. For myself, I believe I have to do my best to think positive, and to choose to think more positive thoughts when I notice I'm not, because positive thinking calls me to action to love myself and the Earth we all live on, including to love you. When we are in a state of love, the immune system is stronger.

What has helped me in the past to encourage more positive thinking, especially through hard and tiring times, was listening to audio programs from teachers such as these:

- Wayne Dyer
- Louise Hay
- Eckhart Tolle

Books like *The Four Agreements* by Don Miguel Ruiz and the works of certain Buddhist authors, among them Pema Chödrön and Thich Nhat Hanh, also help me feel better and stay mentally upbeat. See the Resources section at the back of the book for a list of recommended reading.

All these people are easy to access. They offer free YouTube videos that you can watch at any time, day or night. I enjoy putting their videos on and using them like a meditation practice. Sometimes I may put a video or audio program on in the background while I clean my apartment or make food. You might listen to one before you go to sleep. And then, of course, their products are available as MP3

audios, many from iTunes, that you can listen to on an iPod when you are shopping, exercising, or walking outdoors.

Try listening to some funky music, too. Dance for fun! These kinds of things are good to have around for when you need them. They provide ideas that are soothing and uplifting to the mind and soul.

Positive thinkers embrace the idea of a healthy Earth. When we ourselves are living in the now and in harmony, we resonate with the earth, and the earth responds. Some advanced growers believe that a plant will respond to a gardener who has abundant hands. The more calm, nurturing, kind, loving, conscious, and healthy we are, the more the earth responds, which is great because the earth does produce all our food after all. If the earth is producing healthy food, this helps us to be healthy and helps us to feel and think more positively. It's a win-win situation.

When I remember that life is not hard if I live in the now, I am reminded of plants and how they grow with less resistance, and this reminds me to stay relaxed. Interestingly, I've noticed that when I am relaxed I naturally choose to eat healthier foods.

Here are some affirmations that have helped me and other people to stay mentally positive. Say them aloud several times daily while looking in a mirror or taking a walk. You could also use one or all of them in a row if you are experiencing a negative thought and want to replace it with a positive one.

- *I love my body and appreciate every cell in my body.*
- *I can do it. I am taking the steps that are necessary to live my healthiest life.*
- *Each day I grow and add more nourishment to my life.*
- *I love myself and all is well.*

These are from *Love Your Body* (Hay House, 1989) by Louise Hay, for releasing health problems:[2]

- *My healing is already in process.*
- *I listen with love to my body's messages.*
- *My health is radiant, vibrant, and dynamic now.*
- *I am grateful for my perfect health.*
- *I deserve good health.*

Every aspect of our lifestyle can be a positive experience for us and have a positive impact on Earth.

## Why Are There So Many Chemicals in Our Foods and Products?

Chemicals have taken over our lives because we've accepted their presence in all our products. The Earth Diet lifestyle encompasses everything. Every time we make a purchase, it's like casting a vote. We're telling companies, "Yes, make more of that." That's why each purchase is important. We can either support companies making products with chemicals or eco-focused companies using plant-based ingredients. Eco businesses are usually owned by people with a deep love and understanding of nature who dedicate their lives to sustaining a healthy environment. This way of thinking underlies their choices. Every business operates in a context. My context is a healthy Earth.

Think about where your products come from and who makes them. Is their core value to make money? Or is it to make money by creating products that sustain life on Earth?

In ancient history, the Egyptians made all kinds of natural foods, medicines, and skin-care and body-care products using only organic ingredients, as that was all they had on hand. Somewhere along the line, as the business world started to develop, companies started exploring chemicals that made products cheaper. Most probably didn't know these ingredients were toxic. They thought they were convenient. Today, however, an increasing number of people are getting sick, and we have realized that these supposedly safe chemicals can be linked to our poor health. Eventually these companies will go out of business or will improve their products, making them less harmful to the human body and to Earth. In her book, *The Honest Life*, Jessica Alba says, "The beauty industry has added hundreds of new chemicals to all their cosmetic formulations to improve performance. Now the pressure is on to find safer alternatives for the chemicals we know may work great—but aren't so great for our health. The good news is that a lot of beauty brands are starting to get there."

## On a Budget? Prepare to Save Money and Feel Better

Many people think that living a healing and organic lifestyle can be expensive. It is actually the opposite. Believe it or not, making your own food and products can be 60 percent cheaper than buying them ready-made. The only costs are for the ingredients and your time. Try it for yourself, and do the math! I realize some fast-food restaurants offer entire "meals" for five dollars, and that it is impossible for an organic café to compete with this price because organic produce costs more than genetically modified produce. But . . . a cheap meal is usually made with fast, cheap, fake ingredients, so it really isn't worth having no matter what it costs.

Your health is worth more than that!

Remember that beans, lentils, rice, and potatoes are inexpensive healthy foods, and you can make huge soups and curries with them that can be eaten over a few days for just a few dollars. If you are on tight budget, the most inexpensive Earth Diet recipes are Bean Burgers, Lentil Soup, Vegan Soup, Mushroom Soup, and Vegan Curry. You could also start your own garden and eat from that as much as possible.

If you cannot afford organic yet, go for the types of fresh fruits and vegetables that are grown with fewer pesticides and sprays. If you *can* afford it, I recommend buying organic everything. Why not, if it's better for you and the earth?

We can take inexpensive foods and treatments to help our conditions, which can save us thousands and thousands of dollars in the long run. In *Forks Over Knives: The Cookbook*, Chef Del Sroufe explains, "Any number of diseases—cardiovascular diseases, diabetes, obesity, and more—can be not only prevented, but in many cases *reversed* with the right diet: a whole-foods, plant-based diet. By eating this way, you can cut down on increasingly expensive medical bills and insurance costs. As a bonus, you'll even likely slash your grocery bills, because the healthiest foods, like beans, grains, fruits, and vegetables, also tend to be less expensive than the highly processed foods that are currently making us sick."

Jamie Oliver is another fine chef and health-food revolutionist who agrees that there is no price on our health, and that healthy food is not as expensive as we may think. In his book *Jamie's Dinners,* he says, "It comes down to your perception of value—is it about buying the cheapest thing you can get, or is it about spending a little more and getting something that tastes nicer, smells better and makes you feel good in return?"

## Body-Care Products

Let's break down the issue of lifestyle now to the things we regularly do besides eating, starting with brushing our teeth.

Whenever we brush our teeth we absorb the ingredients in the toothpaste. We should think twice about absorbing what is in regular toothpaste. What is so bad about it? First, it costs more than making your own version. Second, it is full of chemicals, like sodium lauryl sulfates (SLS), artificial flavorings and colorings, parabens, glycerin, fluoride, and more. SLS is one of the worst chemicals found in body-care products. It has been linked to all sorts of health issues, including cancer. Fluoride is also bad.

There are many brands of organic toothpaste to choose from. You can find a selection at most health-food stores and drugstores, and even in regular supermarkets. You can also make your own! Children usually love the taste of homemade toothpaste. I also think it tastes better and less artificial.

I make my own toothpaste using clay, baking soda, coconut oil, salt, and peppermint extract. All the ingredients provide health benefits in addition to cleaning the teeth. The coconut oil has antibacterial properties. The clay, which is tasteless and gives the toothpaste its pasty consistency, draws out toxins from the gums and tongue. Try one of the following two recipes.

# Toothpaste for Three Brushings

## INGREDIENTS:

1 teaspoon baking soda
1 drop peppermint or lemon essential oil
A few drops of water

Mix in a bowl until the paste is formed. Then brush your teeth.

# Three-Month Toothpaste Supply

This recipe makes a little more than one cup of toothpaste. You should be able to make it for under three dollars. You can store it in a jar in the fridge for up to four months, and it will keep in your medicine cabinet at room temperature for 7–14 days.

## INGREDIENTS:

½ cup bentonite clay
⅛ teaspoon salt
2 teaspoons baking soda
⅔ cup water
¼ cup coconut oil
1 teaspoon stevia (optional)
1–4 drops peppermint essential oil

Mix the clay and salt in a bowl. Add the water. Mix well. Add the rest of ingredients. Mix well again until it forms a paste. Store it in a jar with a lid. Every time you go to use it, spoon some onto your toothbrush. Dampen the paste by putting your brush under some gently running water. Brush as usual.

# Tooth Whiteners

Bleaching our teeth white is *not cool*. We are putting so many harmful chemicals on our teeth and in our mouths that seep through to the gums, tongue, and rest of the body that it is scary. Plus whitening your teeth can cost you hundreds of dollars or more. I tried bleaching my teeth once before I knew about the natural alternatives, and it really hurt my teeth and gums. It was not worth me going through that pain.

Now I use baking soda and bentonite clay to whiten my teeth periodically. Both substances are naturally provided by Earth and have health benefits. I alternate between the two, as the baking soda can be abrasive on my teeth and gums. If I start to feel even a tiny sting, I switch to bentonite clay.

**BAKING SODA:** Keep a jar full of it in your bathroom. Spoon ½ teaspoon onto your toothbrush after brushing your teeth. Brush in gentle circular motions, buffing your teeth as if you were going through a car wash. You may want to do this every day for 14 days until your teeth are whiter. Once your teeth are white, stop brushing them with baking soda for a while, until you feel like doing another polish.

**BENTONITE CLAY:** Keep a jar full of it in your bathroom. Spoon ½ teaspoon of it onto your toothbrush after brushing your teeth. Brush in a gentle circular motion on your teeth, just like you do with the baking soda. Do it for a few minutes until you feel like everything is squeaky clean.

## TRY THIS RECIPE:

2 tablespoons of baking soda
2 tablespoons of bentonite clay

Mix them together and store in your bathroom. Put ½ teaspoon on your toothbrush and use it to scrub your teeth. This yields 4 tablespoons of powder, enough for 12 days if you're using ½ teaspoon twice a day.

# Breath Fresheners

Conventional gum is made with chemical ingredients, like aspartame, that are linked to cancer and schizophrenia. No thanks! Instead, use a simple, natural alternative. Most of these are less expensive than purchasing gum.

**CHEW ON:** Ginger slices or a few leaves of parsley, mint, or cilantro. Grow your own. Chew on two leaves of parsley, for instance, before leaving for work in the morning or on your way out the door!

**EAT:** An apple or avocado.

**BRUSH AND GARGLE WITH:** Lemon water (rinse thoroughly afterward so as not to strip your tooth enamel), baking soda, or bentonite clay.

# Deodorant

Stay away from deodorants that contain aluminum. Heavy metals clog the pores and stop sweat from coming out. It is natural for the armpit to perspire toxins, so do not clog it up. Instead:

**CUT:** A lemon in half and wipe it under your armpits.

**PAT:** Your armpits with a little bit of baking soda (about a teaspoonful).

**FIND:** An organic deodorant that uses gentle, plant-based ingredients.

# Perfumes

Use small amounts of essential oils as perfume. Read the labels on the oils first, however, to make sure they can be put directly on the skin. Some great-smelling oils are lavender and rose. A few simple drops of lemon juice can also have you smelling fresh! And you could even add a few drops of pure vanilla extract to your wrists for a vanilla scent.

Stay away from fragrances that are made up of synthetic perfume components. Most commercial scents contain phthalates, which interfere with hormone function and create toxic buildup in the body, thus weakening the immune system and clogging the lymphatic system.

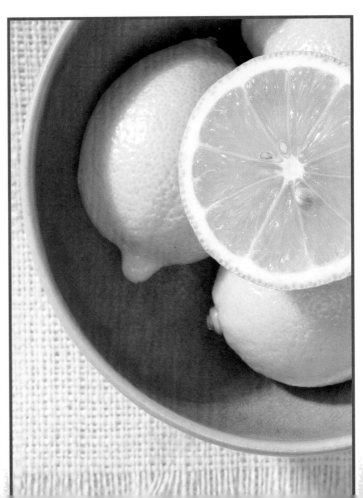

# Moisturizer

Use extra-virgin coconut oil, extra-virgin olive oil, avocado oil, flaxseed oil, aloe vera (the flesh from inside an aloe leaf, or organic aloe vera gel or liquid), or cacao butter. Smooth it onto your skin and rub in.

Here is a recipe for a lush body and face moisturizer.

**3 tablespoons of aloe vera**
**2 tablespoons of coconut oil**
**3–5 drops of essential oil like lavender, mint, or orange (optional)**

Mix together in a bowl and then store in a glass jar or tube. Keep at room temperature or in the fridge. Will last for 3 months. This will yield just under 1/3 cup of face moisturizer. Apply daily or whenever you feel you have dry skin.

# Dry Body Brushing

Use a dry body brush once daily, stroking it in a circular motion, to remove dead skin cells and toxins. Dry brush with a natural-bristled brush. These can be purchased at most health-food stores or on the Earth Diet website. Dry brushing stimulates the body's circulation and lymphatic systems. Many naturopathic doctors use dry brushing to help with bloating because massaging the lymph nodes helps the body shed excess toxins and water as well as improving digestion.

# Sunscreen

**1 cup coconut oil or avocado oil**
**1/2 cup beeswax**
**1/2 cup zinc oxide (zincite)**
**1/2 cup water**

Mix together in a bowl and store in a tube or glass jar. Keep at room temperature. Zincite has UV protection properties, with this sunscreen having SPF 20. The recipe will yield around 2 1/2 cups of sunscreen.

TIPS:

1. You can add vanilla extract or other herbs and oils as you desire.
2. If you want to make a completely vegan sunscreen, you can make it without the beeswax, just add an additional 1/2 cup of oil or shea butter.
3. You could also use straight raspberry seed oil for the highest SPF of about 30–50, carrot seed oil for SPF 30, or sesame seed oil and hemp oil for SPF 4–10, instead of using a recipe.
4. For a higher SPF, you can use hemp oil in this recipe instead of coconut and avocado oil.
5. You can purchase pure zinc oxide from Amazon.com.

Use organic, plant-based, vegan, animal cruelty-free cosmetics. Here are some recipes.

# Mascara

Mascara dates back to ancient Egypt. Most formulas contain the same basic elements: pigmentation, oils, and waxes. But conventional mascaras contain harmful toxic ingredients. You can make your own with ingredients from your local health-food store. The recipe that follows yields just under 2 ounces of mascara.

### INGREDIENTS:

**A clean mascara container that comes with a mascara brush (buy online). If you cannot find one of these, place the mascara in a tiny jam jar and then (carefully!) use a toothpick as the mascara brush. You can also clean out one of the mascara tubes you have at home.**
**1 tablespoon extra-virgin coconut oil or extra-virgin olive oil or avocado oil**
**2 tablespoons aloe vera gel**
**1 1/2 teaspoons beeswax, grated**
**1/4 teaspoon activated charcoal for light black mascara, 1/2 teaspoon activated charcoal for dark black, or 1/2 to one teaspoon of cacao powder for brown. You can usually buy the activated charcoal in capsule form at your health food store. 1/2 teaspoon will be 1–3 capsules depending on their size.**

### DIRECTIONS:

1. Put coconut oil, aloe vera gel, and grated beeswax in a small saucepan over low heat. Stir until the beeswax is completely melted.
2. Add the charcoal to the oil mixture. Stir until completely incorporated. Remove from heat.
3. Pour the mixture into the mascara container. Do this with a funnel or by pouring the mixture into a small plastic bag, and then pushing the mixture into one corner, cutting a small hole in the tip of the bag, and gently squeezing the mixture into the mascara tube.
4. Now store in a fridge or cool place. Once it is cool, it is ready to use!

### TIPS:

If you need more hold to your mascara add more beeswax. Store in the fridge. Keep the lid on tightly so it does not dry out. Replace the mascara tube in 6 months with a fresh new clean one.

# Hair Moisturizing Treatment

Use coconut oil for a hair treatment. Lather hair with oil until saturated, and then let sit for 20 minutes. Wash out with a non-toxic shampoo and conditioner.

You can also treat your hair with bentonite clay, which draws toxins from your hair. I have heard that a lot of people love doing this for a few reasons, including that clay is relaxing for the head, the head feels clean afterward, and the hair feels thicker and more radiant. Some people also like cacao butter treatments, olive oil, banana, and egg.

# Face Masks

Use bentonite clay mask, avocado face mask, or cacao face mask. See the guide for clear skin (p. 175).

## Home Cleaning Products

**LAUNDRY DETERGENT:** If your clothes are washed in chemicals, your skin will absorb them. Make your own detergent using plant-based ingredients. Here is a recipe for a regular load: 1/3 cup liquid pure castile soap, like Dr. Bronner's, and 1 tablespoon of baking soda. For larger or more heavily soiled loads, double it using 2/3 cup of Dr. Bronner's Soap and 2 tablespoons baking soda.

Dr. Bronner's products are 100 percent pure castile soaps and can be purchased all around the world online and in health stores. This natural liquid soap does a great job at washing clothing and even creates a lot of foaming lather. "Pure castile" is your guarantee that you are using real ecological and simple soap, not a complex blend of detergents with a lot of chemicals. This kind of detergent is better for your clothes, your body, and also for Earth, as it has less ecological impact and is biodegradable. Stay away from non-organic laundry detergents as they kill ocean life, including fish and coral.

**AIR FRESHENER:** Combine water, fresh mint, and essential oils in a spray bottle. Try using 2 drops of orange, vanilla, or other essential oils in 2 cups of water. Spray in your home, on carpet, and on furniture.

**COUNTER/ALL-PURPOSE CLEANER:** In a spray bottle, mix 2 cups water, 1 drop tea tree oil, juice of 1/2 lemon, 1/2 tsp pure vanilla extract. Spray on counters and polish clean. To clean dirtier surfaces, add more tea tree oil.

**FLOOR CLEANER:** Mix 8 liters of water in a bucket with 3 drops of tea tree oil and/or 6 drops of pure vanilla extract. Mop the floor as usual.

**FRUIT AND VEGETABLE WASH:** Squeeze the juice of one lemon into two cups of water. Add to a spray bottle and then spray your fruits and vegetables before rinsing them thoroughly, in order to wash off any pesticides or bacteria.

**WATER FILTERS:** I have a water filter on my shower and also on my kitchen tap. This filter alkalizes the water and restores minerals. It also filters chlorine and other heavy metals from the water.

You can get excellent filters from as little as $400 to over $6,000 for an entire house filtration system. Better to drink and shower in clean water than in water with chemicals. I recommend particular filters on my website.

## For Business Owners

There are many ways to make your business more Earth friendly. For example, if you run an office, use organic, biodegradable soaps and paper goods. Put a good filter on your kitchen faucet so there is quality water for everyone to drink. You could also provide a "Recipe of the Month," printing it out and sticking it on the community board to inspire employees to be healthy. Healthy people are more productive.

If you are a restaurant owner, start using cleaner ingredients, especially oils and salts. Use extra-virgin coconut oil for cooking, rather than generic vegetable oils, which are toxic and often genetically modified. Use Himalayan salt or sea salt, as opposed to white table salt, which is toxic. Do not provide Splenda or white sugar; offer local honey, maple syrup, or raw sugar for healthier options. Use as many organic, local, and seasonal ingredients as possible. Also use few, or no, processed ingredients.

# Dangerous Chemicals
## Found in Household and Body-Care Products

Following is a list of chemicals that are found in our household products and body-care products. There have been studies showing that these chemicals are easily absorbed into our bodies, and I believe they contribute to all types of health conditions such as cancer, birth defects, kidney failure, neurological system issues, respiratory issues, brain damage, allergies, rashes, depression, nosebleeds, asthma, breast cancer, immune system issues, reproductive issues, hormone issues, autism, sore throat, eye irritation, headaches, dizziness, fatigue, brain tumors, liver damage, memory loss, obesity, thyroid problems, and more. These chemicals are then put back into our water system and are dangerous to fish, coral reefs, and other sea life.

- Bisphenol A, aka BPA, found in baby toys, baby bottles, sippy cups, some pacifiers, anything plastic labeled #7, canned foods, fast food, bottled-water containers.

- Brominated flame retardants, aka BFRs, *see Flame retardants*.

- Cadmium found in lipsticks and some face paints.

- Ceteareath *see SLS*.

- Chlorine bleach found in laundry detergent, stain removers, and bleach.

- Diethanolamine, aka DEA, found in mascara, concealer, sunless tanning lotion, and conditioner.

- DMDM Hydantoin *see Formaldehyde*.

- GMOs found in some skin-care products might not be listed, or will be listed as Vitamin E, corn, or soy.

- Flame retardants found in nonstick cookware, fabric, water-repellent fabrics, stain-resistant fabrics, foam cushions, mattresses, crib mattresses, kids' pajamas, carpeting, and paints.

- Formaldehyde found in kitchen cabinets, carpeting, mattresses, body washes, shampoos, nail polish and removers, keratin hair straighteners, hair gels, and eyelash glues.

- Fragrance found in household products, perfumes, synthetic musks, home air fresheners.

- Halogenated flame retardants, aka HFRs *see Flame retardants*.

- Hydroquinone found in skin lighteners, moisturizers, hair dyes, and anti-aging creams.

- Imidazolindinyl urea *see Formaldehyde*.

- Lead found in lipsticks and some face paints.

- Mercury found in face paints, mascara, deodorants, and some other eye makeup.

- Mineral oil found in foundations, lotions, cleansers, lipsticks, lip balms, and many other color cosmetics.

- Nickel found in lipsticks and some face paints.

CONTINUED ON NEXT PAGE

- Oleth *see SLS.*

- Optical brighteners found in laundry detergents.

- Parabens found in shower gel, shower lotion, shaving gel, shampoo and conditioner, and cleanser.

- Paraffin found in foundations, moisturizers/lotions, cleansers, lipsticks, lip balms, and many other color cosmetics.

- PEG *see SLS.*

- Perchloroethylene, aka Perc, found in most dry-cleaning formulas and newly dry-cleaned clothes.

- Perfluorinated compounds, aka PFCs, *see Flame retardants.*

- Petrochemicals found in foundations, lotions, cleansers, lipsticks, lip balms, and many other color cosmetics.

- Petroleum jelly found in foundations, lotions, cleansers, lipsticks, lip balms, and many other color cosmetics.

- Phthalates found in nail polishes and anything with the ingredient "fragrance," scented candles, raincoats, flooring, windows, and plastics like shower curtains.

- Propylene glycol found in foundations, moisturizers/lotions, cleansers, lipsticks, lip balms, and many other color cosmetics.

- Quaternium-15 *see Formaldehyde.*

- SLS, aka Sodium Lauryl or Sodium Laureth Sulfate, found in shampoo, bubble bath, soap, and shower gel.

- Toluene found in hair dyes, brow bleaches, skin lightener, anti-aging creams, and nail polish, nail strengtheners, and cuticle treatments.

- Triclocarban *see Triclosan.*

- Triclosan found in antibacterial soap, hand sanitizer, toothpaste, deodorants, mold-resistant and antibacterial fabrics and plastics.

- Triethanolamine, aka TEA.

- Volatile organic compounds, aka VOCs, found in cleaning supplies, air fresheners, pesticides, building materials, paints, furnishings, and anything with a strong scent.

- Xynol *see SLS.*

Do not buy products from companies that are untrustworthy. Some even get away with not listing *all* of the ingredients. It is safer to make your own, or buy from organic companies you trust.

Do not serve any food that is genetically modified. Begin growing your own fresh herbs to add to the food. You can either harm people or help nourish them with your service.

Let your customers know you are becoming more Earth friendly—people are willing to pay more for quality food. Offer meals on the menu that are from the Earth Diet. E-mail us and let us know your ideas, as we would be willing to promote your service to our Earth Diet readers. We love to promote companies—especially restaurants—that are natural. The Earth Diet readers from all around the world are always asking us where they can eat that is local and Earth friendly. We can add your restaurant to the list!

## Growing Your Own Produce

The beauty of gardening is that the food you grow yourself tastes better, as it is so fresh and you literally pluck it straight from your garden and eat it. The taste of fresh-picked ingredients is stronger. The nutrients are also stronger. Think of all the benefits of growing your own and then picking and eating it. You know it was planted from seed, you know what went into it, who touched it, how you got it, what helped that plant to grow, and so on.

Here are some basics. If you are beginning a garden, start with herbs. They are the easiest plants to grow and maintain, and can get you in the habit of tending a garden. Then, if you want to start a "kitchen garden," you could grow the plants on the following list. These are all low maintenance, and will require water once daily unless it rains! The idea is to keep the soil moist but not too wet, and certainly not too dry. You will not need any chemicals to grow these, and it is not common for bugs to eat them.

- Basil
- Chives
- Cilantro
- Dill
- Lavender
- Mint
- Oregano
- Parsley
- Sage
- Tarragon
- Thyme

These herbs can usually last through the winter too, so you will not need to reseed. The parsley and chives can even get snowed on and survive! They are perennial plants!

Take it a step further and grow vegetables—perhaps one tomato plant in a pot or a couple of pea vines. The taste of peas straight out of the pod is awesome and nothing like you would get in a can. Peas and beans are popular plants for children, who love to watch them grow, especially the vines, and then love popping them out of their pods.

Gardening is very relaxing, and many describe it as a meditation. Some people say they connect spiritually to themselves and the earth from watching something grow from seed to fruition. But if the idea of starting from seeds is daunting, remember that you can always start with plants and nurture them from there. Following are some vegetables that bear a great crop of produce and are also easiest to grow and maintain.

- Cucumbers
- Kale
- Lettuce
- Onions
- Peas
- Peppers
- Spinach
- Tomatoes
- Zucchinis

You can also grow your own aloe vera, which is easy to maintain. This succulent can be used in juices or on the skin as a remedy for dryness, burns, sunburn, infections, acne, eczema, and psoriasis. It has remarkable nutritional and healing properties, like being antiviral and antibacterial. It also contains 18 amino acids and high levels of antioxidant vitamins, and stimulates the immune system.

It might be good to ask yourself "What would I like to eat?" and grow the things that you really want to eat! Grow the things that excite you most. Some gardens can produce hundreds of dollars' worth of food in a season. And if you live somewhere like Australia that does not have harsh winters, you can have a garden the entire year. Gardens are good for the economy and your bank account! If you do not feel confident starting on your own, you could be part of a community garden; they are set up for success. Here you can learn from others and maybe even find a mentor who can give you advice—and perhaps also some seeds! Gardeners usually love other gardeners, so you might like to walk through your neighborhood and check out what your neighbors are growing. If it is doing well for them, it will probably do fine for you since you are in the same environment.

If you grew the kitchen garden and had all the herbs to choose from, and then these vegetables, you could make one scrumptious, extremely nutrient-dense salad. I would add avocado and some lemon dressing! My mum has a complete garden at home, and she has also started many of them for her friends. She says it takes a lot of work initially, but is worth it. Protect your plants by building fences if you need to keep animals away. If you do see bugs threatening your crops, here is a recipe for a natural repellent: In a spray bottle, mix 1 entire bulb of minced garlic and 3 cups of water. Shake well and then spray over your plants every day until the bugs are gone.

My own experience of gardening has always been to grow simple things like herbs, tomatoes, pumpkins, and zucchinis. They are easy to maintain and can be grown in a pot or box, like a window box, that is suitable for apartments. Gardening has become more accessible to more people these days, and we can successfully grow in our apartment buildings in smaller pots, or outside in the soil in our yards! We can get a relatively large amount of produce from a small area. I get excited when it is time to harvest, and then I make a delicious meal. It is very fulfilling. Some people have gardens that they completely live off and eat from every day—this is the ideal way to live the Earth Diet!

Remember, gardening can be a lifelong process. There is no need to grow everything all at once; you can start with one thing and grow from there. Make it doable for you. There are online communities that can help. On some websites, you can type in your zip code and find out what seeds are compatible to your area and seasons. *Better Homes and Gardens* offers tips for beginners and advanced gardeners alike.

Note that you can compost your vegetable and fruit scraps, as well as the fiber you get from making juices. This will help accelerate your garden by providing rich soil! If you cannot garden yourself, but want the freshest foods possible, you can rely on your local farmers' market.

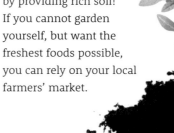

## Fermenting Vegetables

This is a food preserving technique that has been used for hundreds of years, and also comes with many health benefits. It is also a great way to maintain the Earth Diet if you live a busy lifestyle, or have many mouths to feed and want to have food on standby. One of the most famous fermented vegetables is known as sauerkraut, which is fermented cabbage. Fermented vegetables are a powerful natural probiotic that helps with digestion and absorption of nutrients. They can also boost immunity and aid weight loss. It is also a great way to make food using fresh ingredients in the summer, and then store it to eat during the winter.

You can make all types of blends using ingredients like: cabbage, beet, cauliflower, cucumbers, carrots, peppers, and onions.

### THE PROCESS:

1. Chop vegetables into tiny pieces; this allows their liquids to release faster.
2. Mix vegetables with salt and herbs like thyme and oregano.
3. Add water and then place the vegetables into a jar. The water should cover the vegetables by at least half an inch.
4. Keep at room temperature for 3–5 days, and then in the refrigerator indefinitely. This is surprising, but it does truly last for years.

And now that you've begun thinking about where your meals come from and some different ways to use produce, let's move on and talk more about preparations.

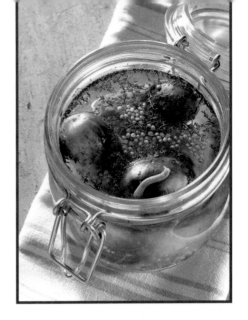

# Pickled Cucumbers

INGREDIENTS:

5 small cucumbers
2 teaspoons mustard seeds
1 tablespoon dill
1 tablespoon salt
1 cup room-temperature water

ACTIONS:

1. Place whole cucumbers and then remainder of the ingredients in a quart-sized jar. The water should cover the cucumbers and the top of liquid should be at least $1/2$ an inch below top of jar, as the water will rise during the fermentation process. You may need more than 1 cup of water, depending on the size of the cucumbers.
2. Cover tightly and store at room temp for 3–5 days before keeping in refrigerator indefinitely.
3. Serve with salads, meat meals, or mix into stir-fries!

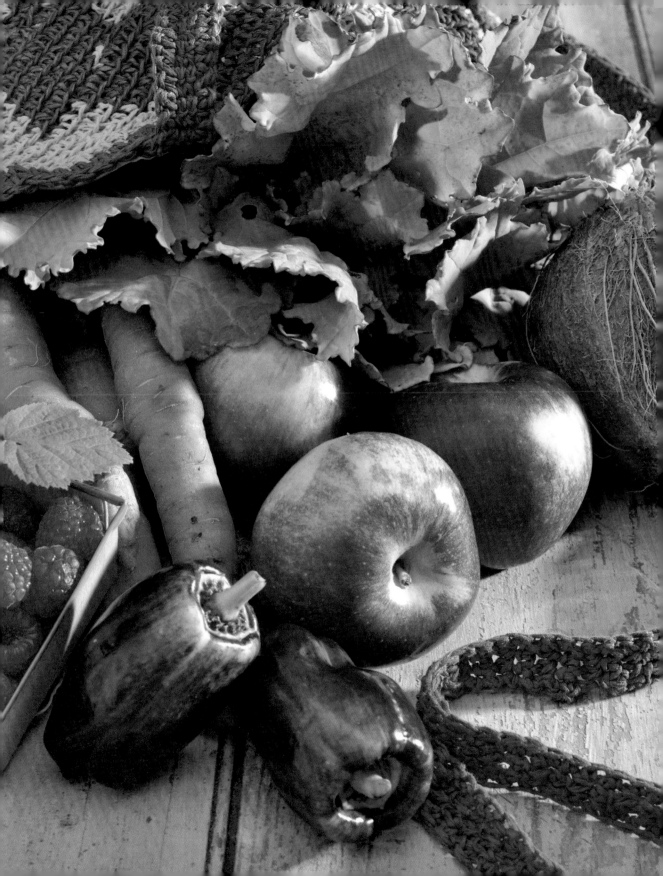

# CHAPTER 4

# Preparations

"All things are ready, if our mind be so."

—William Shakespeare, *Henry V*

We're almost ready to get into the recipe portion of the book. Before we get cooking, however, I'd like to offer you a few words of advice on preparing and modifying the recipes for your personal lifestyle.

As you know, you should choose fresh, organic produce for your meals whenever possible. Organic fruits, nuts, roots, vegetables, herbs, and spices, which by definition are grown chemical free, provide us with the best nutrition. When I refer to "clean foods" or "clean eating," these are the types of foods I am referring to. You should be able to find all these clean ingredients in a local or organic supermarket, a farmers' market, or even online. As you learned in the last chapter, try to grow as much of your own food as possible.

Use the recipes provided in this book as a base for your own cooking, and feel free to modify them to suit your own taste. Make them work for you. The Earth Diet recipes should be considered improvisational. Add more or less of any given ingredient: perhaps more maple syrup as a sweetener or more salt, or more cayenne pepper to make the recipe spicier. Check out the different variations I've suggested at the end of each recipe and get creative. Even with the juices and smoothies, there is room to play. They can be frozen into ice pops and cubes, or even transformed into salad dressings! The Beet Juice makes a great dressing over kale and avocado, and the Strawberry Smoothie makes excellent Strawberry Pops!

Every recipe in this book is loaded with nutrition and designed to provide the body with many health benefits. All are nourishing for the body because they provide essential nutrients, including vitamins and minerals, especially antioxidants, omega fatty acids, amino acids, and the powerful phytonutrients that our bodies need to thrive at the optimum level. Every recipe is nutrient dense and designed to provide us with the maximum nutrition it can contain per bite and per calorie.

## How the Earth Diet Recipes Are Organized

The recipes are divided into sections that specifically focus on juices, smoothies and shakes, teas and waters, raw vegan main dishes, cooked vegan main dishes, main dishes for meat eaters, condiments, and desserts. The vegan recipes use entirely plant-based ingredients: fruits, vegetables, roots, nuts, seeds, herbs, and spices. The recipes for meat eaters use not only beef, poultry, and fish, but also ingredients like eggs. My advice to meat eaters is to prepare your meals from the plant-based recipes at least 70 percent of the time.

I've tried my best to accommodate the needs and desires of every type of eater in this book because I want everyone to be as healthy as possible. Some vegans have expressed anger that I include meat recipes—they believe meat is *never* healthy. I respect their personal choices and agree that people can thrive on an entirely plant-based diet.

I grew up eating meat every day as a child, and I'm accustomed to it. Now that I live the Earth Diet lifestyle, I eat organic and free-range meat, poultry, or fish only once a week. The rest of the time I am eating fruits, vegetables, roots, and the occasional fungi. The majority of my diet is made up of raw fruits, vegetables, juices, and smoothies. This works well for me.

On principle, the Earth Diet encourages a majority raw, vegan, plant-based lifestyle. However, no one gets left behind, and I do have a lot of readers who choose to eat some meat.

## A Few Tips on Modifying the Recipes

Vegans can adapt the meat eaters' recipes for their dietary principles by replacing the suggested meat with additional vegetables. For example, the Beef Stir-Fry is delicious reinvented as a Vegetable Stir-Fry. I also suggest using chunks of eggplant instead of chicken in the recipe for Chicken Nuggets. It easily becomes Eggplant Nuggets. Just try to keep the proportions of primary ingredients relatively constant.

It is very important for those who do eat meat always to choose organic, free-range meat, otherwise you risk contaminating your body with hormones, antibiotics, and GMO ingredients, none of which is acceptable when you're on the Earth Diet.

Of the desserts, some are raw vegan and others are cooked vegan. All of them are strictly vegan *unless* you use raw honey, which is considered an animal product—in this case, the bee. Use maple syrup to keep desserts entirely vegan. Agave, which is both raw and vegan, is not highly recommended, as the manufacturing process it goes through is not as clean as those for pure maple syrup and honey. A clean process means a simple process. For example, plucking an apple from the tree and eating it directly is extremely clean.

When making your desserts and beverages, remember this hierarchy: The best sources of natural sweetness, measured both in terms of which is cleanest and also of which provides the body with the most nutrients, are dates, then raw honey, then maple syrup, then coconut sugar, then stevia, and then agave. Use whichever sweetener feels right for you. All are better than refined white sugar. Raw cane sugar sucked directly out of the cane is also clean.

When juicing, remember that you can use the Earth Diet recipes or make up your own combination of juices. Juice any fruit or vegetable that you feel like drinking!

Simply add the ingredients to your juice machine, pour, and drink to receive a zap of cellular nutrition.

If you have a nut allergy, you can substitute sunflower, pumpkin, or hemp seeds whenever a recipe calls for nuts. Use the same measurements for seeds as you would for nuts.

When juicing, juice the entire fruit or vegetable. For example, if a beet root comes with greens attached, juice the root and greens together. If a carrot comes with leaves attached, juice those, too. If the kale comes with stems, juice those. When juicing apples, you can juice the entire fruit, including the skin. Wash it first to remove dirt and possible bacteria. Always, always wash your produce.

If you prefer to remove apple seeds before juicing, then you can do so. There is a tiny amount of cyanide inside every apple seed. The casing is hard so it usually moves right through your digestive tract and gets eliminated. The question that seems to be endlessly debated is whether or not juicing the seeds increases the risk of exposure. In my opinion, apple seeds are not a big deal for healthy individuals since the amount of the toxin is so slight. Now, if you were to juice an extremely large amount of apples with seeds, it might be unnecessary for your body to have to cope with that. I've never yet met someone who died or got poisoned from drinking raw apple juice.

If you have been diagnosed with cancer or another potentially life-threatening illness, please do your own research, consult your health-care providers and/or refer to the "Specific Foods for Specific Needs" resources section on my website. According to some experts, such as those at the renowned Gerson Institute, where they treat people with cancer using natural methods, there are foods to include or avoid when healing, which include nuts and seeds. They also advocate avoiding high-fat fruits, like avocadoes, and high-sodium vegetables, like cucumbers.[1] See the Recommended Resources section.

## Making a Plan for the Week Ahead

Once a week, perhaps on a Sunday afternoon, get out a pen and paper and make a shopping list for the meals you imagine having in the week ahead. The way I do this is to look at the recipes I plan to use, which include a lemon water, juice, smoothie, probably a piece of raw chocolate or a dessert, a salad, and a cooked dish every day. Sometimes I follow one of the guides in Part III. After I choose the recipes I anticipate making, I pick up the ingredients I need at the grocery store or farmers' market.

As you're thumbing through the recipes, choose the ones that you feel energetically pulled toward. These might be your favorites or ones you haven't tried yet. Follow your bliss.

Your shopping list most likely will include these foods:

- Fruits
- Vegetables
- Legumes (peas, beans, lentils)
- Rice, grains, and brown rice pasta
- Nuts and seeds
- Oils and sweeteners
- Herbs and spices
- Meat (optional)
- Fish (optional)
- Cacao and chocolate (yum)

You can download a more specific checklist-format shopping list on my website, TheEarthDiet.com/BookGift.

Once you know the meals you anticipate making, think about proportions. To save yourself time and effort, you could make a triple portion of a main dish, such as Turmeric Rice. You can have that for dinner one day fresh and then have leftovers for lunch the next day. If there's anything left, you can freeze it and save it for another meal later in the week.

If you have Turmeric Rice for dinner on Sunday, you can also be creative on Monday and wrap ¼ – ½ cup of the rice in a leaf of some kind—romaine lettuce leaves or collard greens work well for this—add a slice or two of avocado, and it makes a nice lunch taco.

Freeze a bunch of juices or smoothies so you always have one handy when you need it. I've been asked how someone can juice when they're not at home near their juice machine. This is one of the ways. Another strategy is to purchase a small, portable hand juicer for a couple of dollars, and leave it in your desk drawer, the kitchen at the office, or your handbag or knapsack. You can become even closer to nature by juicing lemons, oranges, and grapefruits by hand!

You can also freeze a batch of Lemon Water in an ice cube tray so you can then grab one to suck on when you're on the go—or toss several into your portable water bottle in the morning before you go to work. Make your week easy for yourself with simple tricks like this. The Earth Diet is creative!

Make enough salad dressing for the entire week and mix up different salad combinations that get stored in the refrigerator. When it's time to eat your salad, pull one out of the fridge and add dressing, toss it, and voila! Obviously fresh is always best, but when you live a busy lifestyle just do the best you can.

Want to hear a liberating idea? Once a week, I make and store my desserts, too!

For instance, I make up a batch of Chocolate Balls or Cookie Dough Balls (any variation), or Vegan Ice Cream or Cheesecake. I always have Earth Diet desserts in my fridge and freezer ready to eat. This is actually how I cured myself of my compulsive eating habits years ago. For five years I tried to deprive myself of foods that I thought were bad, so I restricted what I ate and felt miserable. Then I gave myself permission to eat whatever I want when I want it as long as it's sourced from the earth.

You might believe this kind of permissiveness means you would eat and eat and never stop eating, but that's not what actually happens. Because you have permission to eat and because the foods you eat are clean and nutrient dense, you find that you stop eating when your body feels fulfilled.

Furthermore, you soon begin knowing exactly what your body is hungry for! For me, this means I sometimes want a salad and sometimes French fries. If I want a salad, I have a salad. If I want dessert, I have dessert. If I want pasta, I have pasta. You get the picture? If you're used to feeling guilty and miserable when you eat, you're going to be amazed.

If there's a food you typically crave—and many people crave sweet, chocolaty foods— you will want to have some on hand, so you don't feel tempted to run out and buy a junk-food snack to satisfy an intense craving. After I make a dessert recipe, I divide it into individual portions (for example, slices of cheesecake) and freeze these for later. Then I can thaw one out any time. They're even good semi-frozen.

The point is: Prepare yourself to eat foods that you love. Food is a big part of our lives, so as a rule don't get out of bed unless you're excited about what you get to eat during the day.

Now, let's look at a few practical considerations for working with the recipes.

## Look for the Nutritional Symbols in the Recipes

All recipes in this book are refined sugar free, dairy free, soy free, corn free, GMO free, preservative free, hormone free, filler free, and additive free. Unless you make the whole-wheat flour Bread Rolls variation instead of the option using rice and buckwheat flour, the recipes are gluten free. Personally, I eat Bread Rolls approximately once a month, and it's easy to have the Gluten-free Rolls if that's the right choice for you.

When you begin working with the Earth Diet recipes, you'll be able to follow the symbols listed below to understand the additional health benefits of each recipe.

 **ANTI-INFLAMMATORY:** This recipe can be used to soothe inflammation because it includes ingredients that allow more blood flow to damaged or irritated tissues. Some recipes with this designation are helpful in soothing symptoms of acne, allergies, cancer, diabetes, heart disease, high blood pressure, celiac disease, obesity, overheating, swelling, tissue damage, and more.

 **ANTIOXIDANT:** This recipe is particularly high in antioxidants, such as vitamin C, vitamin E, and beta-carotene, which are molecules that inhibit the oxidation of other molecules in the body (similar to the way rust destroys metal). Because of how they neutralize free radicals, antioxidants protect cells and repair them from damage. This recipe can increase energy and enhance your mood, and it may be used to help fight conditions such as cancer, arthritis, infections, colds, depression, fatigue, and stress.

 **DETOXIFICATION:** This recipe is so nutrient dense that it has the components necessary to optimize detoxification and elimination. Its ingredients, which may include iron, magnesium, calcium, zinc, and antioxidant vitamins, support the liver to function well and aid in flushing toxins from the intestinal tract, the blood, and the cells. This recipe can be used if your goal is to clean out the body and build a new body with healthier cells.

 **DIGESTIVE HEALTH:** This recipe can be used to help improve the symptoms of irritable bowel syndrome, leaky gut syndrome, constipation, bloating, diarrhea, and cancer, tumors, and ulcers in the digestive tract. What makes a recipe qualify for this designation is that its ingredients are easily digested, and it may be high in fiber, potassium, magnesium, iron, and calcium.

 **HIGH IN PROTEIN:** This recipe is high in protein. Proteins are essential nutrients. They are the building blocks of all the body's tissues because they are packed with amino acids. This recipe is useful for increasing muscle mass, gaining weight, recovering from a workout, or energy maintenance.

**IMMUNE BOOSTING:** This recipe is high in vitamins, minerals, and phytonutrients that support the immune system. Therefore, it can be used to combat any disease, mild or severe, including colds, flus, infections, cancer, and diabetes. When the immune system is strong, it becomes resilient.

 **INCREASE ENERGY:** The ingredients in this recipe boost physical energy. Besides being nutrient-dense, it doesn't require much energy from the body to break them down. This recipe provides instant energy. Some recipes with this designation are considered aphrodisiacs, as their ingredients are libido enhancing. All such recipes are mood elevating.

 **WEIGHT LOSS:** This recipe can be used to accelerate weight loss. It is especially nutrient dense, meaning that while it is high in nutrients, it is also low in calories. This recipe increases the metabolism to the extent that the body can more readily drop excess weight.

*Per-serving nutritional facts on calories, fat, carbohydrates, fiber, and protein are provided for every recipe in this book. This data was acquired through Nutrition Data, a company which calculates its information using USDA standards.*

## Metric Conversions

If you live in a country where people adhere to the metric system, the following chart can help you convert the quantities of ingredients in the Earth Diet recipes from ounces and pounds to grams and kilos.

**USEFUL EQUIVALENTS FOR DRY INGREDIENTS BY WEIGHT**
*(To convert ounces to grams, multiply the number of ounces by 30.)*

| | | |
|---|---|---|
| 1 oz | 1/16 lb | 30 g |
| 4 oz | 1/4 lb | 120 g |
| 8 oz | 1/2 lb | 240 g |
| 12 oz | 3/4 lb | 360 g |
| 16 oz | 1 lb | 480 g |

**USEFUL EQUIVALENTS FOR LENGTH**
*(To convert inches to centimeters, multiply the number of inches by 2.5.)*

| | | | | |
|---|---|---|---|---|
| 1 in | | | 2.5 cm | |
| 6 in | 1/2 ft | | 15 cm | |
| 12 in | 1 ft | | 30 cm | |
| 36 in | 3 ft | 1 yd | 90 cm | |
| 40 in | | | 100 cm | 1 m |

## USEFUL EQUIVALENTS BY VOLUME

| STANDARD CUP | FINE POWDER (E.G., FLOUR) | GRAIN (E.G., RICE) | GRANULAR (E.G., SUGAR) | LIQUID SOLIDS (E.G., BUTTER) | LIQUID (E.G., MILK) |
|---|---|---|---|---|---|
| 1 | 140 g | 150 g | 190 g | 200 g | 240 ml |
| 3/4 | 105 g | 113 g | 143 g | 150 g | 180 ml |
| 2/3 | 93 g | 100 g | 125 g | 133 g | 160 ml |
| 1/2 | 70 g | 75 g | 95 g | 100 g | 120 ml |
| 1/3 | 47 g | 50 g | 63 g | 67 g | 80 ml |
| 1/4 | 35 g | 38 g | 48 g | 50 g | 60 ml |
| 1/8 | 18 g | 19 g | 24 g | 25 g | 30 ml |

## USEFUL EQUIVALENTS FOR LIQUID INGREDIENTS BY VOLUME

| | | | | | |
|---|---|---|---|---|---|
| 1/4 tsp | | | | 1 ml | |
| 1/2 tsp | | | | 2 ml | |
| 1 tsp | | | | 5 ml | |
| 3 tsp | 1 tbsp | | 1/2 fl oz | 15 ml | |
| | 2 tbsp | 1/8 cup | 1 fl oz | 30 ml | |
| | 4 tbsp | 1/4 cup | 2 fl oz | 60 ml | |
| | 5-1/3 tbsp | 1/3 cup | 3 fl oz | 80 ml | |
| | 8 tbsp | 1/2 cup | 4 fl oz | 120 ml | |
| | 10-2/3 tbsp | 2/3 cup | 5 fl oz | 160 ml | |
| | 12 tbsp | 3/4 cup | 6 fl oz | 180 ml | |
| | 16 tbsp | 1 cup | 8 fl oz | 240 ml | |
| | 1 pt | 2 cups | 16 fl oz | 480 ml | |
| | 1 qt | 4 cups | 32 fl oz | 960 ml | |
| | | | 33 fl oz | 1000 ml | 1 l |

## USEFUL EQUIVALENTS FOR COOKING/OVEN TEMPERATURES

| PROCESS | FAHRENHEIT | CELSIUS | GAS MARK |
|---|---|---|---|
| Freeze Water | 32° F | 0° C | |
| Room Temperature | 68° F | 20° C | |
| Boil Water | 212° F | 100° C | |
| Bake | 325° F | 160° C | 3 |
| | 350° F | 180° C | 4 |
| | 375° F | 190° C | 5 |
| | 400° F | 200° C | 6 |
| | 425° F | 220° C | 7 |
| | 450° F | 230° C | 8 |
| Broil | | | Grill |

## Equipment You Will Need

You can make some of the Earth Diet recipes with just a bowl and your hands. Others require tools. The majority can be made with:

**A JUICE MACHINE:** to make juices. Juicers come in different price ranges; and you also might find a perfectly good one being sold used on the Internet, so don't let the price stop you. Stainless steel juice machines have proven to be the best quality. This is your greatest investment in your health and well-being. You can even use a hand juicer to juice citrus fruits for a couple of dollars. They literally work just as well as the expensive machines and it's easier to clean them. Also, review the discussion Juicer vs. Blender that follows this list.

**A FOOD PROCESSOR/BLENDER:** to make smoothies, raw desserts, sauces, and more. Any powerful blender with a reliable motor and sharp, stainless steel blades will work. If you have a strong enough blender you probably won't even need a food processor.

Also, review the discussion Juicer vs. Blender that follows this list.

**A SHARP KNIFE:** to chop and slice your ingredients.

**A CUTTING BOARD:** Bamboo or wood are best. I do not recommend plastic. I prefer bamboo because the plant grows like a weed, is easy to farm and harvest, and therefore is highly sustainable and earth-friendly. If you feel motivated, you can also buy bamboo bowls, plates, and tableware.

For cooked recipes, you'll need:

**QUALITY COOKWARE:** It's important to use cookware that is non-reactive to the foods you cook in it, like stainless steel, ceramic, glass, and lead-free cookware. The best pots for cooking are thick bottomed. Ultimately, slow heating, as you would use when cooking on a fire or over coals, is the most natural form of cooking. Stay away from flimsy pots, or nonstick pots and pans coated with Teflon and other synthetic materials. According to experts I trust, once heated, they spoil food and become toxic.[2]

It also can be helpful to have:

**A FOOD DEHYDRATOR:** to make raw taco bases, pizza bases, crackers, and fruit strips.

**A MORTAR AND PESTLE:** to grind herbs and spices.

## Juicer vs. Blender

In the beginning, many people ask me if they should buy a juice machine or a blender—or both. If you are confused about which products you need to get healthy, here is what I recommend: Start with one. All you really need is a blender to begin with. Then you can at least make smoothies and juices, and start putting a lot more nutrients into your body. After that, your next purchase might be a juice machine so you don't have to strain your smoothies each time you make them into a juice.

The difference between a juice and a smoothie is that juice has no fiber or pulp and smoothies have fiber. The body uses less energy to break down a juice, and it is instant cellular nutrition. A smoothie might be more filling.

Then your next equipment purchase would likely be a dehydrator—or you might buy some seeds to start a garden.

Of the blenders I've seen on the market, I personally enjoy the Vitamix, which is a powerful industrial-quality blender. With it you can make juices, smoothies, and sauces. It can also be used in place of a food processor. A high-speed blender is a practical machine to have in the home unless you live in a remote place with limited electricity. Then your recipes might be more limited. In this case, you could squeeze your fruit juices by hand or with a juice presser. No electricity needed. The Vitamix can make decadent desserts made with plant-based ingredients, whipped cream, raw chocolate, ice cream, smoothies, and more.

My choice of lifestyle is one where I am enjoying life while indulging in all the healthy options and new technology Earth has to offer, so you can see why a good blender is important to me.

I love plant-based ice "cream" way more than ice cream made with dairy. Some ice cream companies make their ice creams with the cheapest ingredients like dairy from cows fed GMOs that produce milk infected by GMOs. After I eat that kind of ice cream, I feel stripped of energy, weird, and unnourished. Thank goodness there are now companies out there making ice creams using organic plant-based ingredients! I love them and I know a lot of other people who do, too. It's wonderful to go to a store like Whole Foods Market and be able to choose from a variety of organic products.

When I make ice cream at my home with my blender and ice cream maker, it's yummy. After I wait excitedly for it to freeze, I top it with the Earth Diet Chocolate Sauce recipe— which is thick and smooth and chocolaty, and only has three ingredients (maple syrup, coconut oil, and cacao powder)—and some toasted nuts. Okay, granted, I could upgrade to a fully raw meal by topping it with raw almonds, but I feel like some crunch, so I roast organic raw almonds. It's a hybrid meal. A delicious ice cream sundae that is also healthy!

Juice machines and blenders are both great technology that can help us to live our healthiest lives, and in the next chapter, we'll look at stocking your pantry so that you're always ready to use them to whip up something nutritious. I offer discounts and recommendations for juice machines and blenders on my website.

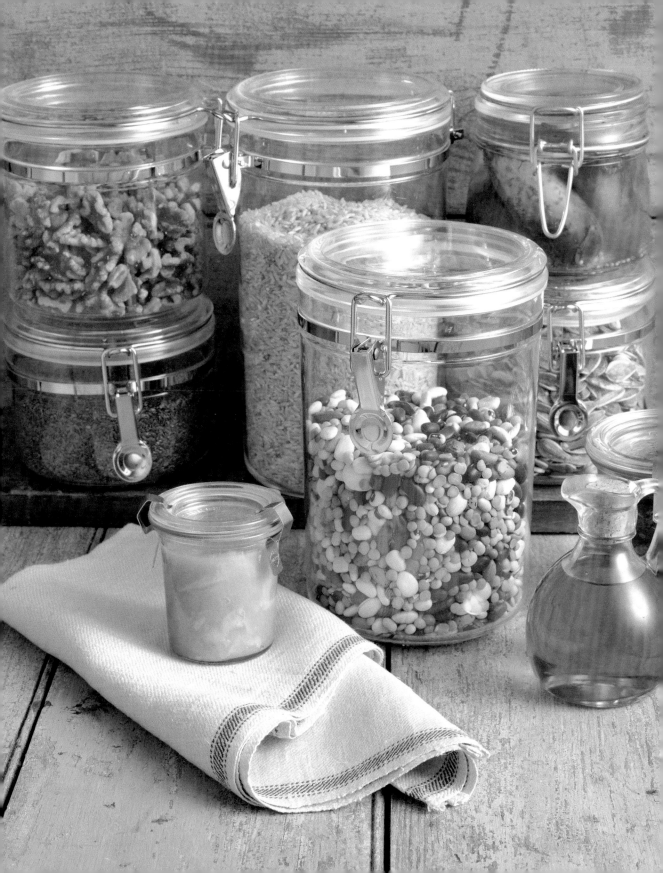

# CHAPTER 5

# Your Pantry

**"As I gave you the green plants,
I give you everything."**

— *Genesis 9:3*

I encourage you to transform your pantry to support a healthy existence. When I mentor someone one on one, the first thing we do is throw out all processed foods and chemical products from their home. Then we go to the supermarket and organic market and stock up on new ingredients and products. We next create an action plan of recipes and natural treatments depending on my client's needs. It is easier to stick to a plan when the environment supports it. If you leave processed foods in your house, it is harder to resist temptation. You won't find processed foods or chemical ingredients in my home anywhere!

## Organic vs. Non-Organic Foods

One of the foremost principles of the Earth Diet is to eat organic food. Organic food is grown without the use of toxic pesticides, herbicides, fungicides, or chemical fertilizers. Organic food is also not genetically modified. For all these reasons, it is "cleaner" than non-organic food.

The best fruits, vegetables, seeds, roots, nuts, and herbs come from plants grown in nutrient-rich soil. Organic farming produces nutrient-rich foods because the methods the farmers use, such as composting, restore the richness of the soil after the crops are harvested. By contrast, non organic produce has been grown with toxic chemicals that deplete the food and soil of nutrients. I always recommend people buy organic. When we eat organic produce, we immediately reduce our chemical exposure.

If, for some reason, you are unable to purchase organic produce, the following list indicates fruits and vegetables grown with the least amount of pesticides.

If a food is labeled *organic*, by regulation, in addition to pesticides, it is not allowed to contain other types of chemicals we want to avoid. Non-organic processed foods, on the other hand, are often filled with artificial sweeteners like aspartame, artificial flavorings and coloring, sodium nitrates, monosodium glutamate (MSG), hormones, antibiotics,

# Lowest
## in pesticides:

1. Onion
2. Avocado
3. Pineapple
4. Cabbage
5. Asparagus
6. Mango
7. Eggplant
8. Kiwifruit
9. Cantaloupe
10. Sweet potato
11. Grapefruit
12. Watermelon
13. Mushrooms

**It is important that you buy and consume only organic fruits and vegetables from the following list, as these tend to be grown with the most pesticides.**

# Highest
## in pesticides:

1. Apples
2. Peaches
3. Nectarines
4. Celery
5. Bell peppers
6. Strawberries
7. Grapes
8. Spinach
9. Lettuce
10. Cucumbers
11. Blueberries
12. Potatoes
13. Kale

preservatives, and additives—giving us more reason to be vigilant.

Even if you do make a point of buying organic, it is still recommended that you wash your fresh produce thoroughly. You can rinse the produce with water alone or make Lemon Water (see p. 100) and clean it in that. The acidity of lemon helps to remove toxins and parasites.

As it is with fruits and vegetables, organic is better for meats. Often, non-organic meat comes from animals that were raised on GMO feeds, including corn and soy, and given hormones to speed their growth and antibiotics to keep them healthy under crowded and unsanitary conditions. All of these toxins remain in non-organic meat; therefore these meats should be avoided.

If you eat meat, eat only meat from free-range birds and animals that are fed organic feed and have never been given hormones or antibiotics. Choose organic produce and meats whenever possible.

## Food Labels

Always use your intuition when reading a label. Many companies are geniuses at marketing and know how to get consumers to buy what they're offering. The other day I was shopping and saw gummy bears labeled "organic." They contained "organic" corn syrup, which experience has taught me isn't possible. As far as I know, nobody makes corn syrup from all-natural, non-GMO corn these days! If you want to learn more about corn syrup, watch the documentary *King Corn* (2007), directed by Aaron Woolf. Look out for tricks like this. If something says "organic" or "natural," check the ingredients list to see just how natural it really is.

Ironically, if a label says "natural flavors," this means it is *not* natural. Something that is natural does not need natural flavors added!

My point is that you should read the labels of everything you eat. Always know what you are eating. As a general rule, if you can't read it, don't eat it! If there are ingredients on a label you cannot pronounce, it means they are very far from being naturally provided by the earth. If any ingredients have numbers, it means they were created in a laboratory and therefore could be extremely toxic. Especially if you see any of the following ingredients listed on a label, stay away from it to ensure that fewer chemicals are being introduced to your body.

## Unacceptable Ingredients in Food Products

The following chemical ingredients (which incorporates Whole Foods' list of unacceptable ingredients) can be extremely toxic and harmful to the human body and have been found to cause many health issues, including cancer, weight gain, depression, addictions, and acne: Acesulfame K (acesulfame potassium), Acetylated esters or mono- and diglycerides, ammonium chloride, added color, artificial colors, artificial flavors and colors, aspartame, azodicarbonamide, benzoates, benzoyl peroxide, BHA (butylated hydroxyanisole), BHT (butylated hydroxytoluene), bleached flour, blue #1, blue #2, bromated flour, brominated vegetable oil (BVO), calcium bromate, calcium disodium EDTA, calcium propionate, calcium saccharin, calcium sorbate, calcium stearoyl-2-lactylate, caprocaprylobehenin, caramel color, carmine, certified colors, corn, corn flour, corn starch, corn syrup, cyclamates, cysteine (l-cysteine), DATEM (diacetyl tartaric and fatty acid esters of mono and diglycerides), dimethylpolysiloxane, dioctyl sodium sulfosuccinate (DSS), dextrose, disodium calcium EDTA, disodium dihydrogen EDTA, disodium guanylate, disodium inosinate, EDTA, enriched flour, ethyl vanillin, ethylene oxide, ethoxyquin, FD&C colors, foie gras, gelatin, glucose, glycerin, GMP (disodium guanylate), hexa-, hepta- and octa esters of sucrose, high fructose corn syrup, hydrogenated fats, IMP (disodium inosinate), irradiated foods, lactylated esters or mono and diglycerides, methylparaben, microparticularized whey protein, MSG (monosodium glutamate), natamycin, nitrates/nitrites, partially hydrogenated oil, polydextrose, potassium benzoate, potassium bisulfite, potassium bromate, potassium metabisulfite, potassium sorbate, propionates, propyl gallate, propylparaben, red #40, saccharin, salt, sodium aluminum sulfate, sodium benzoate, sodium bisulfite, sodium diacetate, sodium glutamate, sodium nitrate/nitrite, sodium propionate, sodium stearoyl-2-lacylate, sodium sulfite, solvent exctracted oils, sorbic acid, sucralose, soy bean, soy bean oil, soy lecithin, sucroglycerides, sucrose polyester, sugar, sulfites (sulfur dioxide), TBHQ (tertiary butylhydroquinone), tetrasodium EDTA, vanillin, vegetable oil, yellow #6, yellow #5 lake.

## Fats and Oils Used in the Earth Diet Recipes

Oils are an important ingredient of the Earth Diet because fats are needed in our bodies for hormone balance and to serve as building blocks for our cells. Only high-quality fats and oils are effective. All fats are not equal. Good fats are those found in avocados, coconut oil, nuts, seeds, fish, and olive oil. The Earth Diet recipes include these healthy fats and oils.

For salads and foods that do not require heating, choose flaxseed oil, extra-virgin olive oil, sunflower oil, and hemp seed oil.

## Top ten nutrient-dense green vegetables:

1. Collard greens
2. Kale
3. Watercress
4. Bok choy
5. Spinach
6. Broccoli
7. Cabbage
8. Brussels sprouts
9. Swiss chard
10. Arugula

## Top ten nutrient-dense nuts and seeds:

1. Sunflower seeds
2. Sesame seeds
3. Flaxseeds
4. Pumpkin seeds
5. Pistachios
6. Pecans
7. Walnuts
8. Almonds
9. Hazelnuts
10. Cashews

## Top ten nutrient-dense vegetables:

1. Radishes
2. Bean sprouts
3. Red peppers
4. Radicchio
5. Turnips
6. Carrots
7. Cauliflower
8. Artichokes
9. Tomatoes
10. Butternut squash

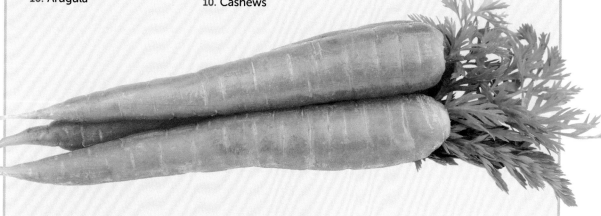

## Top 15 nutrient-dense fruits:

1. Strawberries
2. Blackberries
3. Plums
4. Raspberries
5. Blueberries
6. Papayas
7. Oranges
8. Cantaloupe
9. Kiwis
10. Watermelon
11. Peaches
12. Apples
13. Cherries
14. Pineapples
15. Apricots

For cooking over medium heat, such as light sauteéing, choose sesame oil, pistachio oil, extra-virgin olive oil, and hazelnut oil. For high-heat frying, choose extra-virgin coconut oil, macadamia nut oil, and avocado oil.

Avoid fats that include trans-isomer fatty acids (you've heard these called *trans fats*); hydrogenated or partially hydrogenated oils; and vegetable oils, like canola and unspecified "vegetable" oil as these are also genetically modified.

Avoid deep-fried foods unless you fry them yourself using extra-virgin coconut oil. If you like to eat out, ask your favorite local restaurants to switch to using high-quality oils!

The Earth Diet recipes only use the highest quality oils, those that provide our bodies with excellent nourishment.

## Salts Used in the Earth Diet

Salt is absolutely essential and vital for balancing blood sugar levels, for extracting excess acidity from the cells of the body, for making bones strong, and for nourishing the muscles to prevent them from cramping. There are lots of benefits to salt. But it is important that we eat the right salts.

Although refined white table salt is inexpensive, it can be extremely toxic if it contains an anti-caking agent. Some cheap salts are aluminum based. Others are bleached.

The healthiest salt for the human body is salt in its most whole state, at a point when it is filled with minerals. Choose from rock salt, like pink Himalayan salt, which contains 84 trace minerals, or unprocessed sea salt.

## Getting the Most from Your Produce

If you want to know what fruits, vegetables, nuts, and seeds have the highest amount of nutrients per calories, refer to the lists on the preceding page. These were calculated by evaluating an extensive range of micronutrients, including vitamins, minerals, phytochemicals, and antioxidant capabilities thanks to Whole Foods Market.

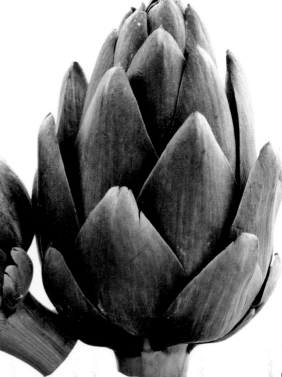

## Stock Your Pantry & Fridge with These Healthy Ingredients

Here is a list of healthy ingredients that are often incorporated into Earth Diet recipes. For each ingredient a description is given that explains three things: its key nutritional facts, some ways people have been using it to improve their well-being, and suggestions of recipes you could make from this book that include it.

The following ingredients might become regulars on your shopping list.

## Almonds and Almond Butter

**KEY NUTRITIONAL FACTS:** high in copper, folate, iron, magnesium, potassium, selenium, vitamin E, zinc, and good fats and protein.

**PEOPLE ARE USING ALMONDS TO:** lose weight, clear acne, lower blood cholesterol and sugar levels, manage heart disease and diabetes, improve focus and memory, uplift mood, and increase energy.

**EARTH DIET RECIPES THAT INCLUDE ALMONDS:** Almond Milk, Almond Butter, Vanilla Shake, Almond Butter Balls, Chocolate Balls, Breakfast Cereal, Vegan Butter, Bean Burgers, Fish and Chips, Burgers, and Chicken Nuggets.

## Apples

**KEY NUTRITIONAL FACTS:** rich in vitamin C and other antioxidants.

**PEOPLE ARE USING APPLES TO:** lose weight, lower cholesterol, and boost metabolism.

**EARTH DIET RECIPES THAT INCLUDE APPLES:** Apple Juice, Beet Juice, Green Juice, Immune-boosting Juice, Apple Cucumber Juice, Slushy, Apple Crumble, and Freezer Pops.

## Apple Cider Vinegar

**KEY NUTRITIONAL FACTS:** high in calcium, magnesium, phosphorus, potassium, and sodium.

**PEOPLE ARE USING APPLE CIDER VINEGAR TO:** make hair shiny, lose weight, aid digestion, relieve constipation, and alkalize the body.

**EARTH DIET RECIPES THAT INCLUDE APPLE CIDER VINEGAR:** Superfood Kale Salad, Vegan Sour Cream, Vegan Butter, Coconut Bacon, Quick Bread, Thai Wraps, and Ketchup. Also, you can drink 1 teaspoon in a cup of water or add it to any of the juices.

## Asparagus

**KEY NUTRITIONAL FACTS:** high in calcium; magnesium; selenium; vitamins A, C, and E; zinc; dietary fiber; and protein.

**PEOPLE ARE USING ASPARAGUS TO:** reduce pain and inflammation, and lose weight.

**EARTH DIET RECIPES THAT INCLUDE ASPARAGUS:** Green Salad and Vegetable Stir-Fry. Also, you can add it to Green Juice and Green Smoothie.

## Avocado and Avocado Oil

**KEY NUTRITIONAL FACTS:** high in potassium; vitamins A, C, E, and K; and good fats.

**PEOPLE ARE USING AVOCADO TO:** lose weight, clear acne, reduce aging, and improve skin health.

**EARTH DIET RECIPES THAT INCLUDE AVOCADO AND AVOCADO OIL: :** Guacamole, Superfood Kale Salad, Chocolate Avocado Mousse, Green Salad, Four-ingredient Green Salad, and Thai Wraps.

## Bananas

**KEY NUTRITIONAL FACTS:** high in vitamins B6 and C, magnesium, potassium, and serotonin.

**PEOPLE ARE USING BANANAS TO:** improve mood, get instant energy, reduce fatigue, reduce insomnia, and sleep soundly.

**EARTH DIET RECIPES THAT INCLUDE BANANAS:** Banana Smoothie, Strawberry Banana Smoothie, Chocolate Banana Smoothie, Chocolate Peanut Butter Smoothie, and Banana Berry Smoothie.

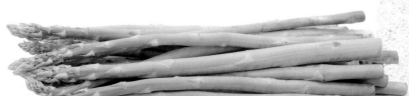

## Beans (Black, Kidney, Lima, Mung, Navy, Pinto)

KEY NUTRITIONAL FACTS: high in B vitamins, iron, folate, lysine, magnesium, potassium, protein.

PEOPLE ARE USING BEANS TO: lower cholesterol; aid digestive health; improve heart health; curb cravings for burgers; and prevent pancreatic, breast, and colon cancer.

EARTH DIET RECIPES THAT INCLUDE BEANS: Bean Burgers and Vegan Curry. You can add them to Green Salad and Vegan Soup.

## Beets

KEY NUTRITIONAL FACTS: high in vitamins A and C, iron, magnesium, calcium, and potassium.

PEOPLE ARE USING BEETS TO: lose weight and accelerate weight loss, lift compacted waste from the bowel walls, boost the immune system, detoxify the blood, purify the blood, cleanse the liver, increase red blood cells to aid in oxygen distribution.

EARTH DIET RECIPES THAT INCLUDE BEETS: Beet Juice. You can add beets to any of the juices, such as Apple Juice, and to salads like Green Salad. You can also add them to Flourless Chocolate Cake.

## Black Pepper

KEY NUTRITIONAL FACTS: high in potassium, calcium, zinc, manganese, iron, magnesium, riboflavin, niacin, and vitamins A and C.

PEOPLE ARE USING BLACK PEPPER TO: improve digestion and absorption of nutrients, reduce flatulence and bloating, fight bacterial growth in the intestines, enhance metabolism, and lose weight.

EARTH DIET RECIPES THAT INCLUDE BLACK PEPPER: Bean Burgers, Burgers, Mashed Potatoes, Cumin Quinoa, Walnut Meat Mixture, and Guacamole. Add it to any recipe to taste.

## Blueberries

KEY NUTRITIONAL FACTS: high in vitamin C and other antioxidants, beta-carotene, fiber, and manganese.

PEOPLE ARE USING BLUEBERRIES TO: lose weight, lower cholesterol, improve brain function, prevent and reduce the symptoms of cancer and other diseases, reduce inflammation, boost immunity, prevent macular degeneration, heal urinary tract infection, and reduce aging.

EARTH DIET RECIPES THAT INCLUDE BLUEBERRIES: Mixed Berry Smoothie, Chia Seed Jam, and Breakfast Cereal. Replace cherries with blueberries in the Raw Cherry Pie recipe for a Blueberry Pie. Also freeze the berries for frozen treats—nature's candy.

## Broccoli

KEY NUTRITIONAL FACTS: high in calcium, folate, vitamins A and C, and fiber.

PEOPLE ARE USING BROCCOLI TO: improve digestion, alkalize the body, prevent cancer and diabetes, improve overall health, boost the immune system, maintain a healthy nervous system, regulate blood pressure, reduce cholesterol and inflammation, and lose weight.

EARTH DIET RECIPES THAT INCLUDE BROCCOLI: Pasta Primavera, Vegetable Stir-Fry, Vegan Soup, and Beef Stir-Fry. Also add it to Green Salad, Green Juice, and Green Smoothie.

## Buckwheat

KEY NUTRITIONAL FACTS: high in chromium; copper; essential amino acids; folate; linoleic acid; magnesium; manganese; protein; and vitamins B1, B2, B3, B5, and E.

PEOPLE ARE USING BUCKWHEAT TO: enhance metabolism, improve liver function and circulation, reduce blood pressure, and replace wheat.

EARTH DIET RECIPES THAT INCLUDE BUCKWHEAT: Mushroom Soup, Gluten-free Rolls, Pancakes, and Quick Bread. You may replace the wheat flour in any recipe with buckwheat to make it gluten free.

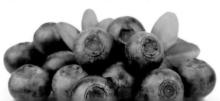

## Cacao (Butter, Powder, and Nibs)

KEY NUTRITIONAL FACTS: high in calcium, copper, iron, magnesium, manganese, oleic acid, potassium, sulfur, zinc, and antioxidants.

PEOPLE ARE USING CACAO TO: increase energy, replace processed chocolate, lose weight, reduce risk of heart attack and stroke, improve brain function, enhance sense of well-being, reduce depression, and improve heart health.

EARTH DIET RECIPES THAT INCLUDE CACAO: Chocolate Balls, Chocolate Avocado Mousse, Chocolate Almond Butter Pie, Chocolate Peanut Butter Cups, Chocolate Milk, Chocolate Smoothie, Chocolate Shake, Chocolate Brownies, Chocolate Block, Three-ingredient Chocolate, Chocolate Sauce, Flourless Chocolate Cake, Cookie Dough Balls, and Freezer Pops.

## Carrots

KEY NUTRITIONAL FACTS: high in calcium; copper; folate; fiber; vitamins B6, C, A; manganese; pantothenic acid; phosphorus; potassium; and thiamin.

PEOPLE ARE USING CARROTS TO: lose weight, improve digestion, boost immunity, prevent heart disease and stroke, reduce aging, aid liver function, and improve eyesight.

EARTH DIET RECIPES THAT INCLUDE CARROTS: Thai Wraps, Beet Juice, Vegetable Stir-Fry, Vegetable Juice, Lentil Soup, Turmeric Rice, Vegan Soup, and Beef Stir-Fry. You can also add it to any of the juices.

## Cashews

KEY NUTRITIONAL FACTS: high in copper, iron, magnesium, potassium, zinc, and antioxidants.

PEOPLE ARE USING CASHEWS TO: improve digestion, regulate blood pressure, and treat cancer and heart disease.

EARTH DIET RECIPES THAT INCLUDE CASHEWS: Cashew Cheese, Raw Cashew Cheesecake, Cookie Dough Balls, Vegan Ice Cream, Vegan Sour Cream, Mushroom Soup, Raw Burgers, Raw Lasagana, Raw Tacos, Raw Pizza, and Zucchini Pasta and Walnut Meat Balls.

## Cauliflower

KEY NUTRITIONAL FACTS: high in folate, magnesium, vitamins C and K.

PEOPLE ARE USING CAULIFLOWER TO: lose weight, reduce inflammation, improve digestion, beat cystic fibrosis, increase energy, boost the immune system, prevent and fight cancer, enhance colon health, relieve aches and pains, and detox.

EARTH DIET RECIPES THAT INCLUDE CAULIFLOWER: Vegetable Stir-Fry, Beef Stir-Fry, and Cauliflower Popcorn. Also, you can eat it raw or add it to juices.

## Cayenne Pepper

KEY NUTRITIONAL FACTS: high in vitamins B6, C, E, K; magnesium; and minerals.

PEOPLE ARE USING CAYENNE PEPPER TO: lose weight, improve circulation and digestion, boost metabolism, internally cleanse, reduce inflammation, soothe arthritis, treat asthma, neutralize acidity, break down the mucus associated with colds and flu, heal stomach ulcers, improve heart health, clear clogged arteries and strengthen the cardiovascular system, prevent heart attacks, heal hemorrhoids, treat prostate cancer, clean the blood, and assist lymphatic health.

EARTH DIET RECIPES THAT INCLUDE CAYENNE PEPPER: Immune-boosting Tea, Weight Loss Tea, Vegan Curry, Beef Stir-Fry, Raw Crackers, Walnut Meat Mixture, Raw Tacos, Raw Lasagna, and Raw Pizza. Also add small quantities to any of the juices, stir-fries, or salads to make them spicy.

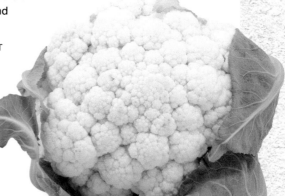

## Celery

KEY NUTRITIONAL FACTS: high in folate; potassium; vitamins B1, B2, B6, C; sodium; and fiber.

PEOPLE ARE USING CELERY TO: lose weight, improve digestion, lower cholesterol and blood pressure, reduce symptoms of arthritis, relieve muscular aches and pains, reduce the frequency and severity of migraines, and replace electrolytes after working out.

EARTH DIET RECIPES THAT INCLUDE CELERY: Green Juice, Celery Juice, Lentil Soup, Vegan Soup, Green Salad, and Guacamole.

## Chamomile

KEY NUTRITIONAL FACTS: high in calcium, folate, magnesium, potassium, and sodium.

PEOPLE ARE USING CHAMOMILE TO: lose weight, improve digestion, treat anxiety, treat depression, prevent insomnia, promote relaxation, reduce allergies, reduce swelling and inflammation, treat diabetes, cleanse the liver, lower blood sugar, treat cuts and wounds, treat colds, alleviate muscle spasms, soothe stomachaches, relieve hemorrhoids, and maintain clear skin.

EARTH DIET RECIPES THAT INCLUDE CHAMOMILE: Relaxation Tea and the skin-moisturizing recipe in the Clear Skin guide. You can also add chamomile to Chocolate Block, or to a bath or hot water for a relaxing soak.

## Cherries

KEY NUTRITIONAL FACTS: high in potassium and vitamins C and A.

PEOPLE ARE USING CHERRIES TO: lose weight, increase energy, boost immunity, improve sleep, improve the ability to focus, relieve arthritis and gout, treat headaches, protect skin from aging due to the effects of ultraviolet radiation, and reduce the risk of heart disease and cancer.

EARTH DIET RECIPES THAT INCLUDE CHERRIES: Cherry Juice and Raw Cherry Pie.

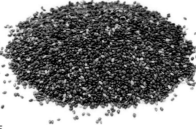

## Chia Seeds

KEY NUTRITIONAL FACTS: high in antioxidants, calcium, copper, iron, magnesium, manganese, niacin, omega-3 fatty acids, zinc, protein, and fiber.

PEOPLE ARE USING CHIA SEEDS TO: increase energy, reduce inflammation, improve digestion, enhance mental performance, lower cholesterol, lose weight, reduce aging, treat thyroid conditions, treat celiac disease, and cleanse the colon.

EARTH DIET RECIPES THAT INCLUDE CHIA SEEDS: Chia Seed Jam and Three-ingredient Chia Seed Cereal. Add to any smoothies.

## Chickpeas (Garbanzo Beans)

KEY NUTRITIONAL FACTS: high in vitamins A, C, K; calcium; choline; folate; magnesium; phosphorus; and potassium.

PEOPLE ARE USING CHICKPEAS TO: boost intestinal health, prevent and heal diabetes, reduce cholesterol, and lose weight.

EARTH DIET RECIPES THAT INCLUDE CHICKPEAS: Hummus, and you can use chickpeas in the Bean Burger for Chickpea Burgers. You can also fry chickpeas in some coconut oil and add salt, cayenne pepper, and turmeric for Chickpea Fries.

## Cilantro (Coriander)

KEY NUTRITIONAL FACTS: high in folate; iron; manganese; vitamins A, B6, C, and K.

PEOPLE ARE USING CILANTRO TO: lose weight, reduce inflammation, improve digestion, detox heavy metals, promote healthy liver function, reduce toxicity, improve bad breath, treat menstrual cramps, and reduce muscle pain.

EARTH DIET RECIPES THAT INCLUDE CILANTRO: Thai Wraps, Green Salad, Four-ingredient Green Salad, Lentil Soup, and Coconut Bacon. Add it to Green Smoothie, Green Juice, or any other juice, like Apple Juice for Apple Cilantro Juice.

## Cinnamon

**KEY NUTRITIONAL FACTS:** high in calcium, iron, manganese, and fiber.

**PEOPLE ARE USING CINNAMON TO:** lose weight, improve digestion, regulate blood sugar, lower cholesterol, treat leukemia and cancer, reduce arthritis pain, and boost brain function.

**EARTH DIET RECIPES THAT INCLUDE CINNAMON:** Apple Pie Juice, Apple Crumble, Breakfast Cereal, and Ketchup. You can also add it to Chocolate Balls and Chocolate Brownies.

## Coconuts and Coconut Oil

**KEY NUTRITIONAL FACTS:** high in calcium, folate, iron, magnesium, phosphorus, potassium, vitamins B5 and C, fiber, and protein.

**PEOPLE ARE USING COCONUT OIL TO:** lose weight, prevent heart disease, lower cholesterol, treat diabetes and chronic fatigue, treat Crohn's disease, treat irritable bowel disorder and other digestive disorders, increase metabolism, promote thyroid function, rejuvenate hair and skin, and prevent aging.

**EARTH DIET RECIPES THAT INCLUDE COCONUT AND COCONUT OIL:** Coconut Milk, Coconut Water, Coconut Bacon, Coconut Basil Sweet Potato Fries, Vegan Curry, Vegan Butter, Chocolate Sauce, Raw Cashew Cheesecake, Raw Cherry Pie, Bean Burgers, and Pasta Primavera. You can also add to smoothies or swallow a teaspoon daily.

## Collard Greens

**KEY NUTRITIONAL FACTS:** high in folate and vitamins A, B, C, and K.

**PEOPLE ARE USING COLLARD GREENS TO:** lose weight, reduce inflammation, improve digestion, prevent and treat cancer, detox, boost immunity, lower cholesterol, support cardiovascular health, prevent and treat diabetes.

**EARTH DIET RECIPES THAT INCLUDE COLLARD GREENS:** Raw Tacos, Green Salad, Thai Wraps, and Raw Burgers. You can also add it to Green Juice and Green Smoothie.

## Cucumber

**KEY NUTRITIONAL FACTS:** high in calcium, magnesium, and potassium.

**PEOPLE ARE USING CUCUMBER TO:** lose weight, improve digestion, boost immunity, hydrate the body, slow aging, reduce inflammation, promote joint health, and relieve arthritis.

**EARTH DIET RECIPES THAT INCLUDE CUCUMBER:** Cucumber Water, Apple Cucumber Juice, Green Salad, Green Juice, and Guacamole.

## Cumin

**KEY NUTRITIONAL FACTS:** high in iron and vitamins A and C.

**PEOPLE ARE USING CUMIN TO:** lose weight, reduce stress, improve digestion and absorption of nutrients, prevent cancer (especially cancer of the colon), relieve headaches, treat infections, boost immunity, increase metabolism, prevent digestive disorders, treat arthritis and diabetes, prevent Alzheimer's disease, prevent macular degeneration, and treat heart disease.

**EARTH DIET RECIPES THAT INCLUDE CUMIN:** Cumin Quinoa, Bean Burgers, Beef Burritos, Raw Crackers, Walnut Meat Mixture, Vegetable Stir-Fry, Pasta Primavera, Lentil Soup, Baked Lamb Chops, Burgers, and Raw Pizza. You can also add cumin to vegetable juices or smoothies.

## Dates

**KEY NUTRITIONAL FACTS:** high in calcium, iron, potassium, magnesium, and phosphorus.

**PEOPLE ARE USING DATES TO:** replace refined sugars, fulfill a candy craving, lose weight, improve diabetes, relieve constipation, heal abdominal cancer, help with intestinal disorders, assist nervous system health, increase energy, help with anemia and fatigue, and improve brain function.

**EARTH DIET RECIPES THAT INCLUDE DATES:** Almond Milk, Seed Milk, Vanilla Shake, Chocolate Shake, and Strawberry Shake. You can also use dates in recipes to replace honey or maple syrup. Add to Breakfast Cereal.

# Eggs

**KEY NUTRITIONAL FACTS:** high in calcium, choline, copper, iodine, iron, magnesium, phosphorus, potassium, selenium, vitamins B and D, zinc, and protein.

**PEOPLE ARE USING EGGS TO:** improve digestion, increase brain function, promote muscular recovery after working out and muscle growth, and lose weight.

**EARTH DIET RECIPES THAT INCLUDE EGGS:** Omelet, Chicken Nuggets, Burgers, Pancakes, and Flourless Chocolate Cake.

# Flaxseeds and Oil

**KEY NUTRITIONAL FACTS:** high in calcium, choline, folate, magnesium, niacin, omega-3 fatty acids, phosphorus, potassium, thiamin, vitamin K, and protein.

**PEOPLE ARE USING FLAXSEEDS AND OIL TO:** lose weight, improve digestion, reduce inflammation, prevent and treat cancer, treat hormonal irregularities, reduce cholesterol and blood lipid levels, reduce blood pressure, prevent osteoporosis, reduce stress, treat ADHD and Tourette's syndrome, and improve mental performance.

**EARTH DIET RECIPES THAT INCLUDE FLAXSEEDS AND OIL:** Superfood Kale Salad, Raw Crackers, Raw Pizza, Flax Egg Alternative, Bean Burgers, and Quick Bread. You can also add flaxseeds or flax oil to juices, smoothies, chocolate balls, and the crust of the Raw Cherry Pie or Raw Cashew Cheesecake.

# Garlic

**KEY NUTRITIONAL FACTS:** high in calcium, iron, magnesium, manganese, potassium, selenium, zinc, and vitamin C.

**PEOPLE ARE USING GARLIC TO:** lose weight, improve digestion, boost immunity, treat colds and flu, cleanse and purify the blood, promote heart health, reduce blood pressure and cholesterol, prevent heart attacks and stroke. It is a natural antibiotic and antifungal.

**EARTH DIET RECIPES THAT INCLUDE GARLIC:** Thai Wraps, Bean Burgers, Beef Burritos, Raw Crackers, Vegan Soup, Coconut Bacon, Lentil Soup, Vegetable Stir-Fry, Green Salad, Immune-boosting Juice, and Immune-boosting Tea. You can also add it to juices like Vegetable Juice or Green Juice.

# Ginger

**KEY NUTRITIONAL FACTS:** high in magnesium and potassium.

**PEOPLE ARE USING GINGER TO:** lose weight, reduce inflammation, boost immunity, improve digestion, cleanse the colon, alleviate motion sickness and morning sickness, fight colds and flus, reduce muscle pain and inflammation, relieve heartburn, and treat migraines and menstrual pain.

**EARTH DIET RECIPES THAT INCLUDE GINGER:** Thai Wraps, Immune-boosting Juice, Apple Cucumber Ginger Juice, Immune-boosting Tea, Weight Loss Tea, Ginger Tea, Green Salad, Lentil Soup, Turmeric Rice, and Salad Dressing.

# Grapefruit

**KEY NUTRITIONAL FACTS:** high in B vitamins, vitamins A and C, potassium, and fiber.

**PEOPLE ARE USING GRAPEFRUIT TO:** lose weight, aid digestion, detox, reduce cellulite, reduce blood pressure and cholesterol levels, prevent cancers, combat colds and flus, and improve eyesight.

**EARTH DIET RECIPES THAT INCLUDE GRAPEFRUIT:** Fat Blaster. Add it to any of the juices or salads, or put it on your cereal.

# Grapes

**KEY NUTRITIONAL FACTS:** high in vitamin K; magnesium; phosphorus; potassium; selenium; and vitamins B1, B2, and C.

**PEOPLE ARE USING GRAPES TO:** boost immunity, aid digestion, lose weight, increase energy, prevent asthma, reduce the frequency and intensity of migraines, and treat indigestion and constipation.

**EARTH DIET RECIPES THAT INCLUDE GRAPES:** Grape Juice. Add it to juices and smoothies.

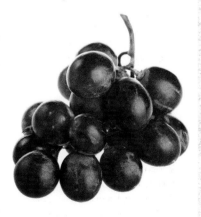

## Green Tea

**KEY NUTRITIONAL FACTS:** high in calcium, vitamins A and C, and protein.

**PEOPLE ARE USING GREEN TEA TO:** boost immunity, lose weight, reduce inflammation, reduce cholesterol, burn fat, detox, prevent cancer and diabetes, prevent stroke and heart disease, and prevent dementia.

**RECIPES THAT INCLUDE GREEN TEA:** Energy Tea. You can add it to Vegan Ice Cream for Green Tea Ice Cream. You can also add it to juices and smoothies. For a stimulating bath, add ½ cup green tea to a bath of hot water.

## Hemp Seeds

**KEY NUTRITIONAL FACTS:** high in essential fatty acids and protein.

**PEOPLE ARE USING HEMP SEEDS TO:** lose weight, improve digestion, and calm the nerves.

**EARTH DIET RECIPES THAT INCLUDE HEMP SEEDS:** Seed Milk, Protein Powder, and Hemp Seed Hummus. You can also use hemp seeds to replace nuts in any recipe.
Add them to Green Salad or Superfood Kale Salad and other salads and soups.

## Honey

**KEY NUTRITIONAL FACTS:** high in glucose, fructose, and antioxidants.

**PEOPLE ARE USING HONEY TO:** improve digestion, boost energy and immunity, lose weight, soothe a sore throat, treat yeast infections and athlete's foot, and reduce blood pressure and arthritis pain.

**EARTH DIET RECIPES THAT INCLUDE HONEY:** Caramel Shrimp, Beef Stir-Fry, Honey Rosemary Chicken, Chia Seed Jam, Almond Butter Balls, and Immune-boosting Tea. You may use honey in any of the desserts in place of maple syrup.

## Kale

**KEY NUTRITIONAL FACTS:** high in calcium; copper; folate; iron; magnesium; manganese; phosphorus; potassium; riboflavin; thiamin; vitamins A, B6, C, and K; fiber; and protein.

**PEOPLE ARE USING KALE TO:** lose weight, boost immunity, improve digestion, prevent colds and flu, strengthen bones, prevent cancers, treat Alzheimer's disease, and boost metabolism.

**EARTH DIET RECIPES THAT INCLUDE KALE:** Superfood Kale Salad, Green Smoothie, Raw Tacos, Raw Burgers, Thai Wraps, and Green Smoothie. Add it to juices, smoothies, and Green Salad.

## Lemons

**KEY NUTRITIONAL FACTS:** high in vitamin C, citric acid, folate, and potassium.

**PEOPLE ARE USING LEMONS TO:** lose weight, increase energy, improve digestion, boost immunity, alkalize the body, prevent and treat cold and flu, treat coughs with phlegm, detoxify, reduce flatulence, alleviate constipation, and reduce blood pressure.

**EARTH DIET RECIPES THAT INCLUDE LEMONS:** Lemon Water, Fat Blaster, Celery Juice, Immune-boosting Tea, Weight Loss Tea, Green Salad, Four-ingredient Green Salad, Salad Dressing, Cashew Cheese, Lentil Soup, and Simple Sage Fish. Add to any juices or smoothies.

## Lentils

**KEY NUTRITIONAL FACTS:** high in calcium, folate, iron, magnesium, vitamins C and K, zinc, and protein.

**PEOPLE ARE USING LENTILS TO:** lower cholesterol, improve digestion, improve heart health, stabilize blood sugar levels, prevent and treat diabetes, treat hypoglycemia, increase energy, oxygenate the blood, and lose weight.

**EARTH DIET RECIPES THAT HAVE LENTILS:** Lentil Soup. You can use lentils in Vegan Curry instead of beans. You can also use lentils in Bean Burgers for Lentil Burgers.

## Lettuce

**KEY NUTRITIONAL FACTS:** rich in thiamin and vitamins A and K.

**PEOPLE ARE USING LETTUCE TO:** lose weight; improve digestion; reduce inflammation; increase energy; strengthen bones; grow red blood cells; maintain healthy skin; improve eyesight; prevent macular degeneration, cancer, Alzheimer's disease, and osteoporosis; treat anemia, and prevent and treat heart disease.

**EARTH DIET RECIPES THAT INCLUDE LETTUCE:** Vegetable Juice, Green Salad, Thai Wraps, and Raw Tacos. You can add lettuce to smoothies and juices.

## Macadamia Nuts

**KEY NUTRITIONAL FACTS:** high in iron, magnesium, omega-3 and omega-6 fatty acids, phosphorus, thiamin, protein, and fiber.

**PEOPLE ARE USING MACADAMIA NUTS TO:** increase energy, regulate cholesterol, prevent heart disease and strokes.

**EARTH DIET RECIPES THAT INCLUDE MACADAMIA NUTS:** Breakfast Cereal. You can use macadamia nuts as a substitute for almonds in the crust for the Raw Cashew Cheesecake recipe. You can also use them in Raw Chocolate Balls and Chocolate Block.

## Maca Powder

**KEY NUTRITIONAL FACTS:** high in copper, iron, manganese, potassium, vitamins B6 and C, and protein.

**PEOPLE ARE USING MACA POWDER TO:** improve digestion, lose weight, increase strength and energy, boost stamina, enhance libido and sexual function, improve memory, reduce stress, and balance hormones.

**EARTH DIET RECIPES THAT INCLUDE MACA POWDER:** Add to Vegan Ice Cream. You can include it in juices and smoothies like the Mixed Berry Smoothie.

## Maple Syrup

**KEY NUTRITIONAL FACTS:** high in copper, iron, manganese, and zinc.

**PEOPLE ARE USING MAPLE SYRUP TO:** increase energy, boost immune system, aid the male reproductive system, assist with heart health, and replace refined sugar.

**EARTH DIET RECIPES THAT INCLUDE MAPLE SYRUP:** Pancakes, Coconut Bacon, Chia Seed Jam, Ketchup, Apple Crumble, Raw Cashew Cheesecake, Cookie Dough Balls, Raw Cherry Pie, Vegan Ice Cream, and Chocolate Sauce. You can also use maple syrup in any of the desserts and as a replacement for honey.

## Mushrooms

**KEY NUTRITIONAL FACTS:** high in fiber; protein; vitamins C, D, and B6; thiamin; riboflavin; niacin; potassium; copper; and selenium.

**PEOPLE ARE USING MUSHROOMS TO:** lose weight, boost immunity, replace meat, boost the immune system, lower cholesterol, assist in the regulation of diabetes, and reduce the risk of breast and prostate cancer.

**EARTH DIET RECIPES THAT INCLUDE MUSHROOMS:** Mushroom Soup. Add mushrooms to Green Salad, Beef Stir-Fry, Vegetable Stir-Fry, and Superfood Kale Salad.

## Nutritional Yeast

**KEY NUTRITIONAL FACTS:** high in B12, magnesium, selenium, sodium, folate, niacin, zinc, amino acids, and iron.

**PEOPLE ARE USING NUTRITIONAL YEAST TO:** lose weight, improve digestive health, replace cheese, relax the body, increase energy.

**EARTH DIET RECIPES THAT INCLUDE NUTRITIONAL YEAST:** Superfood Kale Salad, Cashew Cheese, Bean Burgers, Cauliflower Popcorn, and Mac 'n' Cheese. Add it to Mashed Potatoes and Omelet for cheesy flavor.

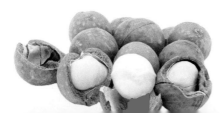

## Olive Oil

KEY NUTRITIONAL FACTS: high in vitamin E, beta-carotene, and omega-9 fatty acid.

PEOPLE ARE USING OLIVE OIL TO: reduce inflammation, lose weight, lower cholesterol and high blood pressure, prevent many types of cancer, strengthen bones, and aid cognitive function.

EARTH DIET RECIPES THAT INCLUDE OLIVE OIL: Green Salad, Salad Dressing, Lentil Soup, Walnut Meat Mixture, Raw Lasagna, Raw Burgers, Roast Chicken, Hummus, Vegan Butter, Cauliflower Popcorn, Zucchini Pasta with Walnut Meat Balls, and Zucchini Pasta with Pesto.

## Onions

KEY NUTRITIONAL FACTS: high in vitamins A, E, and C; folate; choline; calcium; magnesium; phosphorus; potassium.

PEOPLE ARE USING ONIONS TO: boost immunity, lose weight, increase energy, reduce inflammation, alkalize the body, facilitate detoxification, prevent cancer, reduce aches and pains in the body, improve prostate health, ease arthritis, improve symptoms of asthma, improve breathing, help with cardiovascular disease, reduce high blood pressure, prevent heart attack and stroke, improve stomach and digestive health, prevent bowel cancer, maintain firm skin, and prevent osteoporosis.

EARTH DIET RECIPES THAT INCLUDE ONIONS: Vegetable Stir-Fry, Beef Stir-Fry, Vegan Curry, Vegan Soup, Lentil Soup, Turmeric Rice, Beef Burritos, Raw Crackers, Raw Pizza, Green Salad, Coconut Bacon, Bean Burgers, and Pasta Primavera.

## Oranges

KEY NUTRITIONAL FACTS: high in vitamin C, thiamin, folate, potassium, calcium, and fiber.

PEOPLE ARE USING ORANGES TO: boost immunity; increase energy; lose weight; prevent and treat cold and flu; alleviate constipation; regulate blood pressure; prevent cancer and heart disease; purify the blood; aid in teeth and bone strength; prevent and treat diseases like asthma, bronchitis, pneumonia, and arthritis.

EARTH DIET RECIPES THAT INCLUDE ORANGES: Orange Juice, Fat Blaster, Orange Sorbet, Freezer Pops, Thai Wraps, and Mixed Berry Smoothie.

## Parsley

KEY NUTRITIONAL FACTS: high in protein; vitamins E, A, C, K, and B6; thiamin; riboflavin; niacin; phosphorus; zinc; pantothenic acid; fiber; folate; calcium; magnesium; potassium; copper; and manganese.

PEOPLE ARE USING PARSLEY TO: lose weight, increase energy, improve digestion, boost immunity, aid in optimal health, prevent cold and flu, heal ear infections, prevent heart disease and some cancers, treat arthritis.

EARTH DIET RECIPES THAT INCLUDE PARSLEY: Four-ingredient Green Salad, Coconut Bacon, and Mushroom Soup. You can also add parsley to any smoothie or juice like Vegetable Juice.

## Peanuts

KEY NUTRITIONAL FACTS: high in protein, calcium, niacin, folate, vitamins E and B6, manganese, magnesium, phosphorus, potassium, copper, and omega-6 fatty acid.

PEOPLE ARE USING PEANUTS TO: increase energy; gain weight; lower blood pressure and cholesterol; improve blood flow to the brain; prevent many cancers, heart disease, Alzheimer's disease, and age-related cognitive issues; and improve the strength of teeth and bones.

EARTH DIET RECIPES THAT INCLUDE PEANUTS: Chocolate Peanut Butter Cups, Peanut Butter, and Protein Powder.

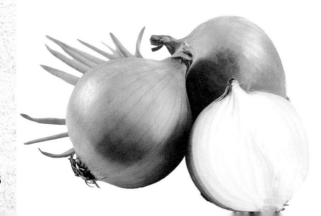

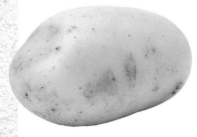

## Potatoes

**KEY NUTRITIONAL FACTS:** high in vitamins C, B1, B3, B6; potassium; iron; phosphorus; magnesium; folate; insoluble fiber; protein; and antioxidants.

**PEOPLE ARE USING POTATOES TO:** prevent colon cancer, prevent and heal diabetes, and help maintain colon health and good digestion.

**EARTH DIET RECIPES THAT INCLUDE POTATOES:** Mashed Potatoes, French Fries, Vegan Curry, Fish and Chips, and Vegan Soup.

## Pumpkin Seeds

**KEY NUTRITIONAL FACTS:** high in zinc, magnesium, and omega-3 fats.

**PEOPLE ARE USING PUMPKIN SEEDS TO:** boost immunity, get high amounts of protein, replace nuts, improve heart health, help with diabetes, get better sleep, and provide an anti-inflammatory for the body.

**EARTH DIET RECIPES THAT INCLUDE PUMPKIN SEEDS:** Protein Powder and Seed Milk. Add them to any smoothies, juices, soups, curries and salads. You can also use pumpkin seeds for Raw Chocolate Balls. Use pumpkin seeds to replace nuts in any recipe.

## Quinoa

**KEY NUTRITIONAL FACTS:** high in insoluble fiber, protein, and antioxidants.

**PEOPLE ARE USING QUINOA TO:** lose weight, help maintain colon health and good digestion.

**EARTH DIET RECIPES THAT INCLUDE QUINOA:** Cumin Quinoa. You can serve it with curries, soup, or stir-fries.

## Rice (Brown)

**KEY NUTRITIONAL FACTS:** high in fiber, manganese, magnesium, selenium, and omega-3 and omega-6 fatty acids.

**PEOPLE ARE USING RICE TO:** improve digestion; increase energy; lower cholesterol; assist the nervous system; satisfy appetite and aid in weight loss; reduce the risk of insulin resistance and metabolic syndrome; strengthen bones and teeth; and reduce risk of heart attack, stroke, and breast cancer.

**EARTH DIET RECIPES THAT INCLUDE RICE:** Turmeric Rice, Mac 'n' Cheese, Pancakes, Gluten-free Rolls, Quick Bread, and Pasta Primavera. You can serve rice with curries, soups, and stir-fries.

## Sage

**KEY NUTRITIONAL FACTS:** high in fiber; vitamins A, C, E, K, and B6; calcium; thiamin; copper; folate; iron; manganese; and magnesium.

**PEOPLE ARE USING SAGE TO:** lose weight, boost immunity, increase energy, increase memory and brain function, treat Alzheimer's disease, reduce the severity of inflammatory conditions like rheumatoid arthritis, heal bronchial asthma and atherosclerosis, and to treat symptoms of menopause, such as hot flashes and night sweats.

**EARTH DIET RECIPES THAT INCLUDE SAGE:** Simple Sage Fish, Walnut Meat Mixture, Raw Tacos, Raw Pizza, Raw Lasagna, Bean Burgers, Vegan Curry, Vegan Soup, Lentil Soup, Burgers, Roast Chicken, and Baked Crusted Salmon. You can add sage to salads and meat dishes.

## Salt (Unrefined Himalayan Salt or Sea Salt)

**KEY NUTRITIONAL FACTS:** high in essential trace minerals.

**PEOPLE ARE USING SALT TO:** improve digestion, lose weight, regulate water content, promote healthy blood-sugar levels, prevent muscle cramping, and promote sinus health.

**EARTH DIET RECIPES THAT INCLUDE SALT:** Superfood Kale Salad, Raw Chocolate Balls, Chicken Nuggets, Cashew Cheese, Coconut Bacon, Hummus, Mac 'n' Cheese, Mushroom Soup, and Walnut Meat Mixture.

## Sesame Seeds

KEY NUTRITIONAL FACTS: high in vitamin B1, calcium, copper, dietary fiber, iron, magnesium, manganese, and phosphorus.

PEOPLE ARE USING SESAME SEEDS TO: lose weight, heal and prevent diabetes, aid vascular and respiratory health, ease asthma, lower blood pressure, prevent stroke, aid with good sleeping, help with menopause, prevent and heal colon cancer, assist with bone health, and ease arthritis.

EARTH DIET RECIPES THAT INCLUDE SESAME SEEDS: Tahini, Raw Crackers, Hummus, Vegetable Stir-Fry, and Beef Stir-Fry. You can also add it to Green Salad, Superfood Kale Salad, soups, and curries.

## Spinach

KEY NUTRITIONAL FACTS: high in protein; fiber; vitamins A, C, E, K, and B6; niacin; zinc; thiamin; riboflavin; folate; calcium; iron; magnesium; phosphorus; potassium; copper; and manganese.

PEOPLE ARE USING SPINACH TO: lose weight, increase energy, promote digestive health, boost the immune system, maintain good blood-sugar levels, prevent and relieve constipation, reduce the risk of cataracts and macular degeneration, promote bone strength and reduce the risk of osteoporosis, reduce the risk of atherosclerosis and stroke, and maintain healthy nervous system and brain function.

EARTH DIET RECIPES THAT INCLUDE SPINACH: Green Spinach Juice, Raw Lasagna, Zucchini Pasta with Pesto, Green Salad, and Vegetable Stir-Fry.

## Sprouts

KEY NUTRITIONAL FACTS: high in protein; fiber; vitamins A, C, and K; calcium; niacin; thiamin; riboflavin; folate; pantothenic acid; iron; magnesium; phosphorus; copper; zinc; and manganese.

PEOPLE ARE USING SPROUTS TO: boost the immune system; increase energy; lose weight; aid in the generation of new cells in the body; increase strength of teeth and bones; lower cholesterol; control hot flashes, menopause, PMS, and fibrocystic breast tumors; and treat pancreatic, colon, and leukemia cancers.

EARTH DIET RECIPES THAT INCLUDE SPROUTS: Thai Wraps and Green Salad. Add to smoothies and juices.

## Strawberries

KEY NUTRITIONAL FACTS: high in antioxidants, vitamin C, manganese, fiber, folate, and potassium.

PEOPLE ARE USING STRAWBERRIES TO: aid weight loss, boost immunity, increase energy, improve heart health, help with cancer, and improve inflammatory bowel problems.

EARTH DIET RECIPES THAT INCLUDE STRAWBERRIES: Strawberry Smoothie, Strawberry Milk, Strawberry Shake, Mixed Berry Smoothie, Slushy, and Chia Seed Jam.

## Sunflower Seeds

KEY NUTRITIONAL FACTS: high in vitamin E and potassium.

PEOPLE ARE USING SUNFLOWER SEEDS TO: improve digestive health, boost immune system, increase energy, raise serotonin levels in the brain, boost nerve function, reduce inflammation, and relieve arthritis symptoms.

EARTH DIET RECIPES THAT INCLUDE SUNFLOWER SEEDS: Superfood Kale Salad, Seed Milk, Raw Crackers, and Raw Pizza. You can add it to salads, soups, and stir-fries and use to replace nuts.

## Sweet Potatoes

KEY NUTRITIONAL FACTS: high in vitamins A, C, E, and B6 and manganese.

PEOPLE ARE USING SWEET POTATOES TO: achieve blood health, heart health, good brain function, and lower blood pressure; prevent and heal cancer; improve vision; prevent and heal macular degeneration; promote healthy hair and skin.

EARTH DIET RECIPES THAT INCLUDE SWEET POTATOES: Coconut Basil Sweet Potato Fries, Vegan Curry, and Vegan Soup. You can also juice them, and boil them to make Mashed Sweet Potato Fries.

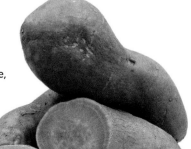

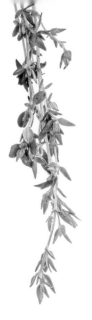

## Tomatoes

**KEY NUTRITIONAL FACTS:** high in antioxidants; vitamins C, A, and K; and potassium.

**PEOPLE ARE USING TOMATOES TO:** lose weight, boost the immune system, improve heart health, improve brain function, increase energy, and support healthy cardiovascular function.

**EARTH DIET RECIPES THAT INCLUDE TOMATOES:** Vegetable Juice, Raw Tomato Sauce, Ketchup, Walnut Meat Mixture, Raw Burgers, Raw Tacos, Raw Pizza, Raw Lasagna, and Zucchini Pasta and Walnut Meat Balls.

## Turmeric

**KEY NUTRITIONAL FACTS:** high in fiber, vitamins C and B6, iron, potassium, and magnesium.

**PEOPLE ARE USING TURMERIC TO:** boost immune system; lose weight; reduce inflammation; detoxify the liver; be an antiseptic and antibacterial agent; disinfect cuts and burns; reduce the size of cancerous tumors; reduce the risk of childhood leukemia; aid in weight loss; and treat inflammatory diseases like arthritis, rheumatoid arthritis, and psoriasis.

**EARTH DIET RECIPES THAT INCLUDE TURMERIC:** Turmeric Rice, Weight Loss Tea, Immune-boosting Juice, Immune-boosting Tea, Cumin Quinoa, Baked Lamb Chops, Chicken Nuggets, Fish and Chips, Vegetable Stir-Fry, Raw Crackers, and Raw Pizza.

## Thyme

**KEY NUTRITIONAL FACTS:** high in fiber; vitamins A, C, E, and K; thiamin; magnesium; zinc; copper; folate; calcium; iron; and manganese.

**PEOPLE ARE USING THYME TO:** lose weight; improve digestion; boost the immune system; help control heart rate and blood pressure; reduce the effects of stress; treat coughs, bronchitis, and chest congestion; kill a range of bacteria and fungus in the body; help prevent some cancers.

**EARTH DIET RECIPES THAT INCLUDE THYME:** Walnut Meat Mixture, Raw Burgers, Raw Lasagna, Vegetable Stir-Fry, Baked Crusted Salmon, Roast Chicken, Mac 'n' Cheese, and Lentil Soup. You can also add thyme to stir-fries and salads.

## Vanilla Beans and Pure Vanilla Extract

**KEY NUTRITIONAL FACTS:** high in manganese and omega-3 and omega-6 fatty acids.

**PEOPLE ARE USING VANILLA TO:** lose weight, increase energy, boost immunity, alleviate nausea, lose weight, reduce anxiety and stress, and assist with the regulation of menstruation cycles.

**EARTH DIET RECIPES THAT INCLUDE VANILLA:** Vegan Ice Cream, Vanilla Shake, Vanilla Smoothie, Raw Cashew Cheesecake, Cookie Dough Balls, Raw Cherry Pie, and Pancakes.

## Walnuts

**KEY NUTRITIONAL FACTS:** high in protein and omega-3 fatty acid.

**PEOPLE ARE USING WALNUTS TO:** increase energy, lose weight, consume a high-protein source, help heal prostate cancer, improve brain health, improve the health of sperm, promote the growth of thicker, shinier hair, stimulate the brain, and increase energy.

**EARTH DIET RECIPES THAT INCLUDE WALNUTS:** Walnut Meat Mixture, Raw Tacos, Raw Lasagna, Raw Pizza, Raw Burgers, Zucchini Pasta with Pesto, Zucchini Pasta with Walnut Meat Balls, Baked Lamb Chops, Baked Crusted Salmon, and Raw Cupcakes. Also use walnuts in Raw Chocolate Balls and Chocolate Brownies.

# CHAPTER 6

# Your First Steps

**"A journey of a thousand miles begins with a single step."**

—Lao-Tzu

We can all do something to upgrade our health and take it to the next level. At the very basic level, every person should be receiving some kind of nutrition daily. Just make one improvement each day, anything that moves you closer toward good health. Remember we never arrive at a place where we're "done." Health is a constant, ongoing process. So just start!

If you feel tired and in pain, try focusing on the positive aspects of your life, however small. You can completely transform your health and your body, and it starts the very moment you choose.

One of the first steps you should take if you want to be healthier is drinking a glass of Lemon Water first thing in the morning to rehydrate and alkalize your body. Besides promoting cellular health, straight away this sets a precedent for the day: "This is going to be a healthy day! I'm on the right track!"

Probably one of the best things you could do for your brain is drink a lot of fresh, clean water. When we don't get enough water, we're just not as sharp as we would be otherwise. Ideally, we should be drinking half our body weight in ounces every day. For example, a 140-pound woman or man would need to drink 70 ounces per day. Chronic dehydration can be a contributing factor in constipation, asthma, diabetes, headaches, high cholesterol, bladder and kidney problems, and even weight gain. Sometimes when we think we're hungry, we're actually dehydrated!

Since the Earth Diet is about "nutrition in, toxins out," an obvious first step is to cut as many junk foods from your diet as possible. That will make you feel better immediately. Seriously! You see, for every processed food you skip, you're going to substitute something more nutrient-rich. Your body gains more energy because it doesn't have to expend effort synthetizing chemicals and digesting weird GMO ingredients.

If you ever catch yourself wondering, *Is this an Earth Diet food?* then think about how natural the food is and what process it had to go through to get put into your hands. If it is in its natural whole and raw state, well, that is as close to the earth as you can get! If you can pick the food right from the tree it grew on, then it will provide your body with immense nutrition. If it is packaged, contains over 20 blended ingredients, including refined sugars and GMO ingredients, then it is absolutely not approved on the Earth Diet. Some people call the Earth Diet the diet that nature, or God, intended for us.

For people who are not yet ready to make a full-time commitment to the Earth Diet, I also can recommend mono eating for one meal a day. *Mono eating* is very simple. It means making a meal out of only one type of food. As an example, you could eat nothing but:

- Bananas for breakfast
- Mangoes for lunch
- Avocados for dinner
- Watermelon for an entire day

The primary benefit of eating mono meals is that it is very easy for the body to digest the food and receive a high dose of nutrients from them. Great benefits of this style of eating are that it usually results in accelerated weight loss, detoxification, boosted immunity, and increased energy. You could try eating mono meals once a week or once a month to give your digestive system a little bit of relief. Or if you splurge one night on something you're not too proud of eating, either a poor food choice or a special indulgence, a mono meal or two can put you right back on track.

Another important way to begin transforming your diet is by juicing once a day—this can mean everything from hand squeezing one orange to making the recipe for Beet Juice (see page 77) in a juice machine. In my opinion, juicing is essential. I recommend that every human being on Earth have at least one fresh, organic juice every day for the rest of his or her life.

When we juice, we provide our bodies many vitamins, minerals, and phytonutrients, and this gives us tons of energy. Juicing is different than eating whole foods, because when we juice we receive nutrition without fiber, so the nutrients are absorbed into our bloodstream, and then by the cells, more quickly than when we eat whole foods. Like mono eating, juicing boosts our energy and accelerates weight loss. Try drinking one juice per day for five days and see how you feel.

And even simpler than mono meals and juicing or using a recipe, you can simply use one ingredient, for example chewing on a cilantro leaf, and get nutrition from that. These are other quick and simple ways to get nutrition from basic ingredients:

- Chew and suck on 1 teaspoon of green tea leaves, then swallow.
- Add ¼ teaspoon of turmeric powder to your mouth, drink some water, and swallow.
- Chew, suck, and allow herb leafs to dissolve in your mouth, including oregano, parsley, and sage.
- Chew on ¼ teaspoon fennel leaves.
- Chew on one garlic clove and then swallow, or just swallow an entire clove.

And remember instead of chewing them, you can make any of these into a tea by simply boiling water and adding the ingredient to it.

## Cleaning Out the Cupboards

Like Old Mother Hubbard, go to the cupboard in your kitchen, but instead of fetching a bone for your dog, take a garbage bag with you and fill it up with the processed, chemical-laden foods you have stored there. Then do the same in your refrigerator and freezer. If throwing away food seems wasteful to you, you could give those foods to a local food bank.

Fill up your kitchen cabinets and fridge with the foods I recommended in the previous chapter, Your Pantry, as these are needed for the Earth Diet recipes that are coming up in Part II.

When you're done with food and beverages, turn your attention to improving the quality of your household cleaning products, such as you would find under the kitchen or bathroom sink. Replace toxic products with organic equivalents. You'll find recipes for homemade supplies in Chapter 3.

Finally, do the same with your body-care products, such as your deodorant, moisturizer, shampoos, and conditioners. In Chapter 3, I give you recipes for earth-friendly, human-friendly toiletries.

By removing toxins from your environment, and eliminating temptation, you've already made it much easier to create a new habit of living a healthy lifestyle.

Looking back on the period when I began keeping my blog, I remember being focused entirely on the changes I was making in my eating habits. Then it clicked! I should change everything I was putting on my skin or spraying in my house, since the skin is the biggest organ in the body and highly absorbent. Now everything I use is organic. I make many of my own products. Others I buy. It is now second nature to live as I do.

## When You're Ready to Go Deeper

Depending on what kind of person you are and what's motivating you to make a change in your lifestyle, you might want to transition quickly into the Earth Diet, like I did when I was facing life-threatening health issues. Or you might want to transition gradually so that your body adapts without undue stress. Either way is good, for as the Buddha said, "A jug fills drop by drop."[1]

Especially when individuals are highly toxic to begin, it is common for them to experience detoxification symptoms as they transition to a more alkaline, plant-based diet. For guidance on managing those symptoms, such as headaches or flulike achiness, please refer to Chapter 2. Other people are not as accustomed to getting as much fiber as they do from fruits and vegetables, so it takes a short period of adjustment. You might find you need to go to the bathroom more often. Fiber increases the speed with which food moves through the digestive tract. Fortunately, discomfort will soon subside. If you experience the opposite effect—constipation—you may want to up your water intake.

A gradual transition can be facilitated by replacing one meal a day for one week and then increasing the number of meals, or by substituting one healthy food for one toxic food. In my case, processed chocolate was my food addiction. I "had to" have it every day. I switched that out for raw chocolate balls. That took a big burden off my health. Then I stopped buying French fries in fast-food restaurants. I switched those out for homemade fries made with sweet potatoes and coconut oil.

If you're ready for a quick start and full-on experience, dive right on into the recipes in the next section. Remember to listen to your body and what you're craving. I eat whenever I feel like it and when I am hungry. But I always eat healthy versions of the dishes I'm craving. Some days I am hungrier than others. I listen to my body and eat when I need to.

I eat a bit of everything. I allow myself to eat only if I am excited about the meal or my body is craving it. I eat all of the recipes in this book! I also drink fresh juice daily, for cellular nutrition. Seventy percent of my diet is raw, and 30 percent is cooked. If you want to incorporate more raw foods into your diet, good recipes to try are the Green Juice and the Superfood Kale Salad. I eat until I am fulfilled and feeling nourished. I love this quote that has been attributed to Hippocrates: "Everything in excess is opposed to nature."[2]

# Five Tips to
# Make It Easier to Transition

1. At the beginning of every Earth Diet recipe, I tell you how long it takes to make it. As a time-saving measure, you can rely upon the recipes that can be made in ten minutes or less.

2. I also recommend making a few recipes in larger quantities once weekly and keeping them in the freezer or fridge so you can have pre-made meals to eat throughout the week. For example, the Chocolate Balls, raw desserts, and Hummus are easy to store and take with you to work or travel.

3. One of the Earth Diet health coaches suggested to a client who was working a 50-hour-a-week schedule that she could prepare seven 16-ounce juices and store them in the freezer. Every morning she could grab one and take it with her to the office. By the time she was ready to drink it, the juice would be thawed.

4. Grow a parsley or cilantro plant to hold yourself accountable to your new lifestyle. Taking responsibility for watering and nurturing this plant will open up your heart and cause you to appreciate your food on a new level. By doing this, you become connected on a daily basis to nature. You learn that you can use it for many benefits besides as a seasoning for your cooking and raw juices, including chewing a piece before you go out as a breath freshener.

5. Say thank you every time you eat. Gratitude improves the digestion and will increase your overall sense of well-being.

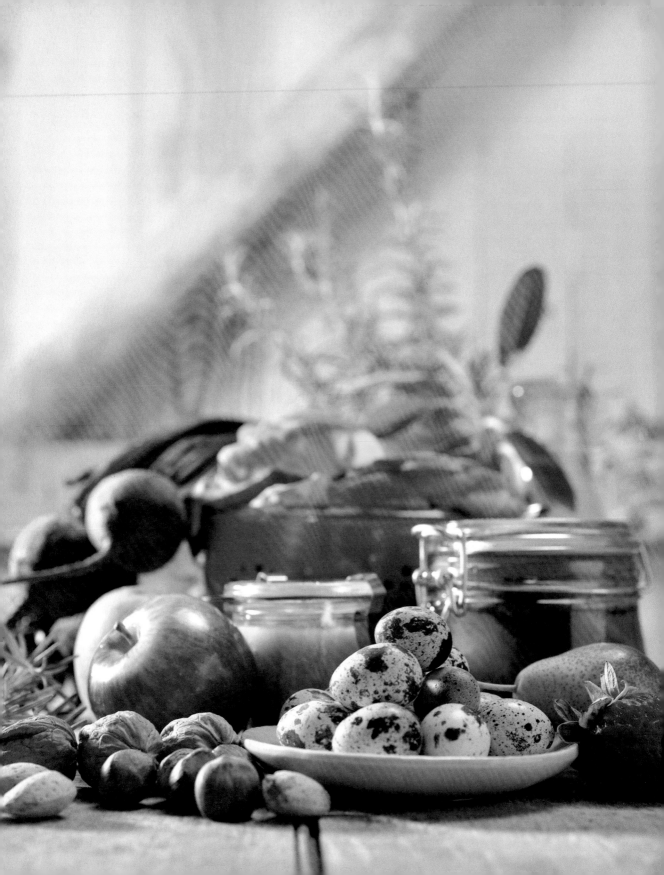

# PART II

# The Earth Diet Recipes

"Simplicity is the ultimate sophistication."
— Leonardo da Vinci

CHAPTER 7

# Juices

Juicing is the quickest
way for us to get a
high dose of nutrition
immediately.

Green Juice, Fat Blaster, and Beet Juice

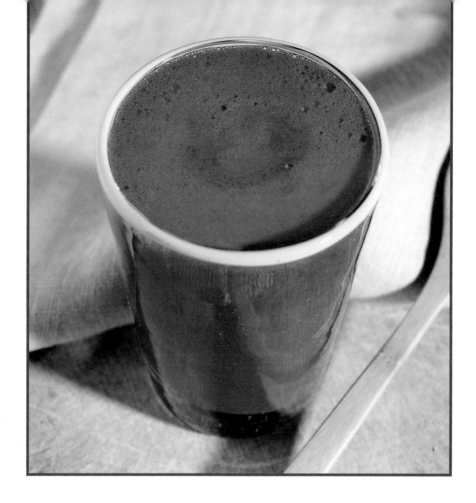

# Beet Juice

*Total time:* **10 minutes** | *Serves* **1**

### INGREDIENTS:

1 small beet
2 red apples
3 carrots

### ACTIONS:

1. Put all the ingredients in the juicer.
2. Juice and drink.

### TIPS:

1. Add 3 celery stalks for extra nutrients.
2. Add 1 small lemon with rind for extra nutrients.
3. Replace the apples with more carrots or celery for 100% vegetable juice.

### VARIATION:

Add 1 two-inch piece ginger for Spicy Beet Juice.

*Calories:* **257** | *Total Fat:* **1g**
*Carbohydrate:* **64g** | *Dietary Fiber:* **1g**
*Protein:* **5g**

### HEALTH BENEFITS:

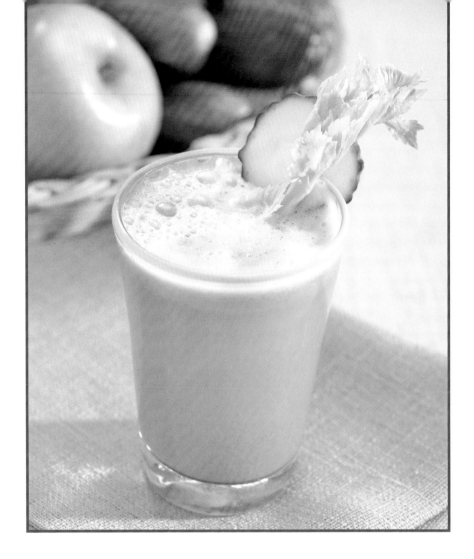

# Green Juice

*Total time:* **10 minutes** | *Serves* **1**

### INGREDIENTS:

1 cucumber
2 green apples
3 celery stalks

### ACTIONS:

1. Put all the ingredients in the juicer.
2. Juice and drink.

### TIP:

Add 1 small lemon with rind for extra nutrients including vitamin C.

### VARIATIONS:

1. Add 1 cup of kale for Green Kale Juice.
2. Add 1 cup of spinach for Green Spinach Juice.
3. Add 1 cup of parsley for Green Parsley Juice.

*Calories:* **210** | *Total Fat:* **1g**
*Carbohydrate:* **54g** | *Dietary Fiber:* **1g**
*Protein:* **4g**

### HEALTH BENEFITS:

# Immune-boosting Juice

*Total time:* **10 minutes**  |  *Serves* **1**

### INGREDIENTS:

**2-inch chunk of turmeric root (If you cannot find fresh turmeric root, use 1 teaspoon turmeric powder.)**
**1 garlic clove**
**1-inch chunk of ginger**
**3 red or green apples**

### ACTIONS:

1. Put all the ingredients in the juicer.
2. Juice and drink.

### TIPS:

Add any of the following or all of them to the Immune-boosting Juice.

1. ½ cup parsley
2. ½ cup spinach
3. ½ cup cilantro
4. 2 celery stalks
5. 2 carrots
6. 1 pear
7. You can replace the apples with 12 carrots to make it a pure vegetable juice.

*Calories:* **248**  |  *Total Fat:* **1g**
*Carbohydrate:* **66g**  |  *Dietary Fiber:* **1g**
*Protein:* **2g**

### HEALTH BENEFITS:

# Cherry Juice

*Total time:* **15 minutes**  |  *Serves* **1**

This juice requires you to pit the cherries. You can either treat it as a meditation or buy a cherry pitter and save time.

### INGREDIENTS:

**4 cups pitted cherries**

### ACTIONS:

1. Put the cherries in the juicer.
2. Juice and drink.

### TIP:

Add ¼ cup of water if you would like to make a less-concentrated flavor and increase the volume of your juice.

### VARIATION:

Add 1 apple to make Cherry Apple Juice.

*Calories:* **340**  |  *Total Fat:* **1g**
*Carbohydrate:* **87g**  |  *Dietary Fiber:* **1g**
*Protein:* **7g**

### HEALTH BENEFITS:

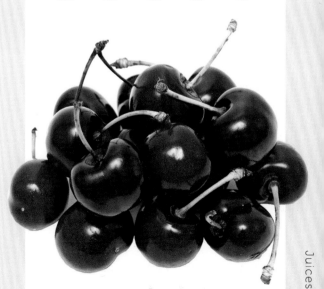

# Orange Juice

*Total time:* **10 minutes** | *Serves* **1**

INGREDIENTS:

**4 oranges, peeled**

ACTIONS:

1. Put the oranges in the juicer.
2. Juice and drink.

TIP:

Add 1 lemon with rind for a boost of vitamin C.

*Calories:* **155** | *Total Fat:* **1g**
*Carbohydrate:* **36g** | *Dietary Fiber:* **1g**
*Protein:* **2g**

# Apple Juice

*Total time:* **10 minutes** | *Serves* **1**

INGREDIENTS:

**4 red or green apples**

ACTIONS:

1. Put the apples in the juicer.
2. Juice and drink.

VARIATIONS:

1. Add ½ teaspoon cinnamon powder for Apple Pie Juice.
2. Add 1 lemon with rind for a vitamin C boost and Lemon Apple Juice.

*Calories:* **315** | *Total Fat:* **1g**
*Carbohydrate:* **85g** | *Dietary Fiber:* **1g**
*Protein:* **2g**

HEALTH BENEFITS:

# Fat Blaster

*Total time:* **10 minutes** | *Serves* **1**

Did you know that grapefruit contains 88–95 percent limonene, a powerful agent for blasting fat and cellulite away?

INGREDIENTS:

**2 oranges, peeled**
**1 grapefruit, peeled**
**1 lemon with rind**

ACTIONS:

1. Put all the ingredients in the juicer.
2. Juice and drink.

TIPS:

1. To feel even closer to nature, for this one you can squeeze the fruit by hand, discarding the rind. If you hand squeeze the lemon but still want to include the rind, you can use a vegetable peeler and scrape off some rind into the juice, then stir.
2. Add more oranges if you would like it sweeter.

VARIATION:

Add a dash of cayenne pepper for Hot Fat Blaster.

*Calories:* **175** | *Total Fat:* **1g**
*Carbohydrate:* **50g** | *Dietary Fiber:* **1g**
*Protein:* **5g**

HEALTH BENEFITS:

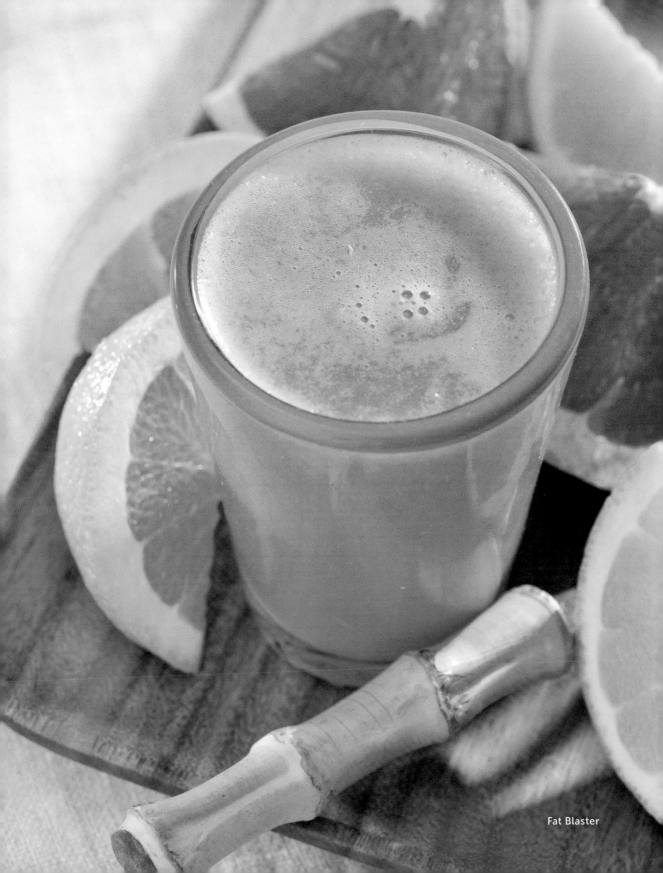

Fat Blaster

# Apple Cucumber Ginger Juice

*Total time:* **10 minutes** | *Serves* **1**

### INGREDIENTS:

**2 large green apples**
**1 large cucumber**
**1-inch piece ginger**

### ACTIONS:

1. Put all the ingredients in the juicer.
2. Juice and drink.

### TIPS:

1. Add 1 lemon with rind for a vitamin C boost.
2. This is a juice for cleansing and supporting the gall bladder.

*Calories:* **203** | *Total Fat:* **1g**
*Carbohydrate:* **53g** | *Dietary Fiber:* **1g**
*Protein:* **3g**

### HEALTH BENEFITS:

ANTI-INFLAM. | WEIGHT LOSS | DETOX | AO | IMMUNE BOOST

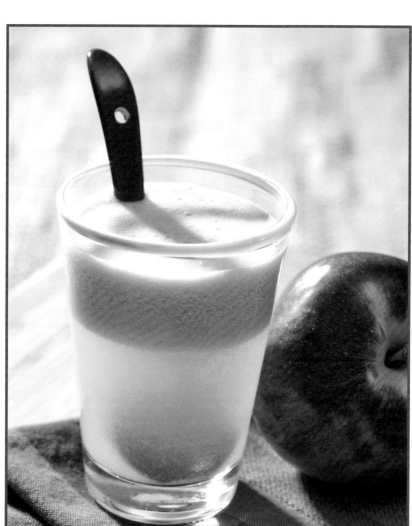

# Vegetable Juice

*Total time:* **10 minutes** | *Serves* **1**

This juice works well for people with diabetes because the ingredients are non-starchy, and it is a great way to get the vitamins and minerals your body needs while preventing an excessive blood sugar response.

## INGREDIENTS:

**1 head lettuce (any kind works well, including iceberg or red leaf, or even kale)**
**2 medium-sized tomatoes**
**3 carrots**

## ACTIONS:

1. Put all ingredients in the juicer.
2. Juice and drink.

## TIPS:

Add one or all of the following to the juice.

1. 1 red bell pepper
2. 1 green bell pepper
3. 1 yellow bell pepper
4. 2 parsnips
5. 1 small purple onion
6. ½ teaspoon salt
7. ½ teaspoon cracked black pepper
8. 1 cucumber

## VARIATION:

Add ¼ teaspoon cayenne pepper (more if you like it spicy) for Spicy Vegetable Juice.

*Calories:* **125** | *Total Fat:* **1g**
*Carbohydrate:* **25g** | *Dietary Fiber:* **1g**
*Protein:* **9g**

## HEALTH BENEFITS:

# Celery Juice

*Total time:* **10 minutes** | *Serves* **1**

## INGREDIENTS:

**½ bunch of celery (6–8 stalks)**
**1 lemon with rind**

## ACTIONS:

1. Put the celery and lemon in the juicer.
2. Juice and drink.

## TIPS:

1. Add 1 apple or more to make it sweeter.
2. Add ½ inch piece ginger for added health benefits.

*Calories:* **26** | *Total Fat:* **1g**
*Carbohydrate:* **11g** | *Dietary Fiber:* **1g**
*Protein:* **3g**

## HEALTH BENEFITS:

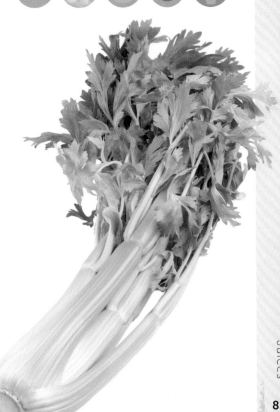

# CHAPTER 8

# Milks
# and
# Milkshakes

# Almond Milk

*Total time:* **10 minutes** | *Serves* **4**

Use this recipe as your base, and then you can make it into anything you like, including Chocolate Milk and Strawberry Milk!

## INGREDIENTS:

**1 cup almonds, skins included**
**4 cups water**
**4 seedless dates**

## ACTIONS:

1. Put all ingredients in the blender.
2. Mix together until a smooth milky consistency is achieved. Drink.

## TIPS:

1. For a creamier and smoother almond milk, soak your almonds for four hours, until the skin is soft; then you can pop the almonds right out of their skins before blending. The only reason the recipe above does not call for the almonds to be removed from their skins is so you can make milk in less than ten minutes.
2. Instead of dates, try substituting 1–2 tablespoons of raw honey or maple syrup.
3. Any kind of raw nut can be substituted for the almonds in this recipe.
4. If you have a nut allergy, use sunflower seeds, pumpkin seeds, flaxseeds, or hemp seeds instead of almonds. See Seed Milk (p. 86).
5. Use cold water for chilled milk.
6. Add 3 cups of ice for thicker, cooler milk.
7. Add a dash of salt, for extra flavor.

## VARIATIONS:

1. Add ½ teaspoon pure vanilla extract and ⅛ teaspoon salt for Vanilla Almond Milk.
2. Add 2 teaspoons (or more, to taste) of cacao powder for Chocolate Almond Milk.
3. Add ½ cup strawberries for Strawberry Almond Milk.
4. Use cashews instead of almonds for Cashew Milk.
5. Use Brazil nuts instead of almonds for Brazil Nut Milk.
6. Use macadamias instead of almonds for Macadamia Nut Milk.
7. Use ¾ cup rice for Rice Milk.
8. Use oats for Oat Milk.

*Calories:* **226** | *Total Fat:* **18g**
*Carbohydrate:* **24g** | *Dietary Fiber:* **6g**
*Protein:* **8g**

## HEALTH BENEFITS:

PROTEIN  AO  ENERGY  DH  ANTI-INFLAM.

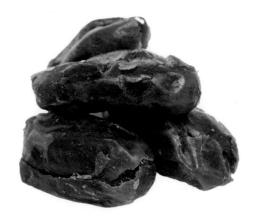

Milks and Milkshakes

85

# Coconut Milk

*Total time:* **10 minutes** | *Serves* **1**

## INGREDIENTS:

**1 fresh coconut, both the liquid and the meat**

## ACTIONS:

1. Make a hole in the coconut. Here is the easiest way: On one end of every coconut you'll see three darker circles together. One of the holes will be softer than the others. Poke through this hole with a screwdriver or a sharp kitchen utensil, like a thin knife or a metal chopstick.
2. Drain the liquid from coconut into a blender.
3. Crack open the coconut with a hammer, then scrape out the white coconut pulp flesh inside and add to the blender.
4. Blend on high speed until a smooth creamy coconut milk is achieved.

## TIP:

Add a dash of salt for added flavor.

## VARIATIONS:

1. Add ½ teaspoon of pure vanilla extract for Vanilla Coconut Milk.
2. Add 1 teaspoon cacao powder, for Chocolate Coconut Milk.
3. Add ½ cup strawberries, for Strawberry Coconut Milk.

*Calories:* **374** | *Total Fat:* **28g**
*Carbohydrate:* **30g** | *Dietary Fiber:* **12g**
*Protein:* **6g**

## HEALTH BENEFITS:

# Seed Milk

*Total time:* **10 minutes** | *Serves* **4**

This is a great recipe for people with nut allergies or people who are nut free.

## INGREDIENTS:

**1 cup sunflower seeds**
**4 cups water**
**4 seedless dates**

## ACTIONS:

1. Put all ingredients in the blender.
2. Mix together until a smooth, milky consistency is achieved.

## TIPS:

1. Instead of dates, try substituting 1–2 tablespoons of raw honey or maple syrup.
2. Use cold water for chilled milk.
3. Add 3 cups ice for thicker, cooler milk.
4. Add a dash of salt, for extra flavor.

## VARIATIONS:

1. Add 1 teaspoon pure vanilla extract and ⅛ teaspoon salt for Vanilla Seed Milk.
2. Add 2 teaspoons cacao powder for Chocolate Seed Milk.
3. Add ½ cup strawberries for Strawberry Seed Milk.
4. Use hemp seeds instead of sunflower seeds for Hemp Seed Milk.
5. Use pumpkin seeds instead of sunflower seeds for Pumpkin Seed Milk.

*Calories:* **271** | *Total Fat:* **18g**
*Carbohydrate:* **25g** | *Dietary Fiber:* **5g**
*Protein:* **8g**

## HEALTH BENEFITS:

# Vanilla Shake

*Total time:* **10 minutes**  |  *Serves* **1**

## INGREDIENTS:

1 cup Almond Milk (see p. 85) or
   Seed Milk (see p. 86)
1 ½ teaspoons pure vanilla extract
3 seedless dates
½ cup ice

## ACTIONS:

1. Put all the ingredients in the blender.
2. Mix until well combined.

## TIPS:

1. To be even closer to nature, substitute
   the seeds of 1 vanilla bean for the
   vanilla extract. You can put the entire
   bean into the recipe as long as the
   blender is powerful enough that it
   won't leave any chunks of the pod.
2. Instead of dates, use 2–3 tablespoons
   maple syrup (or raw honey).
3. Add ⅛ teaspoon salt, for enhanced
   flavor.
4. Add 2 cups crushed ice, to transform
   your shake into a smoothie.
5. Add your favorite superfoods, such
   as maca powder, acai, cacao powder,
   coconut oil, chia seeds, ginseng, green
   tea, or greens powder; or any fruits,
   such as strawberries, blueberries, or
   raspberries.

## VARIATION:

Add 1 banana for Banana Shake.

*Calories:* **490**  |  *Total Fat:* **18g**
*Carbohydrate:* **81g**  |  *Dietary Fiber:* **11g**
*Protein:* **9g**

## HEALTH BENEFITS:

# Chocolate Shake

*Total time:* **10 minutes**  |  *Serves* **1**

## INGREDIENTS:

1 cup Almond Milk (see p. 85) or
   Seed Milk (see p. 86)
2 teaspoons cacao powder
4 seedless dates
½ cup ice

## ACTIONS:

1. Put all ingredients in the blender.
2. Mix until well combined.

## TIPS:

1. Instead of dates use 2 teaspoons maple
   syrup (or raw honey).
2. Add ½ teaspoon pure vanilla extract.
3. Add ⅛ teaspoon salt, for enhanced
   flavor.
4. Add 1–2 bananas or 2 cups crushed ice,
   to transform your shake into
   a smoothie.

*Calories:* **489**  |  *Total Fat:* **19g**
*Carbohydrate:* **84g**  |  *Dietary Fiber:* **13g**
*Protein:* **11g**

## HEALTH BENEFITS:

# Strawberry Shake

*Total time:* **10 minutes** | *Serves* **1**

### INGREDIENTS:

1 cup **Almond Milk (see p. 85)**
  **or Seed Milk (see p. 86)**
½ cup **strawberries**
3 **seedless dates**
½ cup **ice**

### ACTIONS:

1. Put all ingredients in the blender.
2. Mix until well combined.

### TIPS:

1. Instead of dates use 2–3 tablespoons maple syrup (or raw honey).
2. Add 1 teaspoon of pure vanilla extract for enhanced flavor.
3. Add ¼ teaspoon salt, for enhanced flavor.
4. Freeze the strawberries to make a thicker, cooler shake.
5. Make the shake a smoothie by adding another ½ cup of strawberries and ½ cup ice.

### VARIATION:

Add 1–2 bananas for a Strawberry-Banana Smoothie.

*Calories:* **494** | *Total Fat:* **18g**
*Carbohydrate:* **85g** | *Dietary Fiber:* **12g**
*Protein:* **10g**

### HEALTH BENEFITS:

 AO  ENERGY  WEIGHT LOSS  PROTEIN  DH

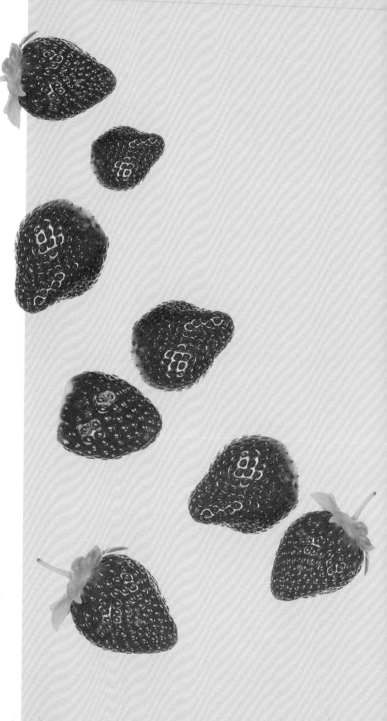

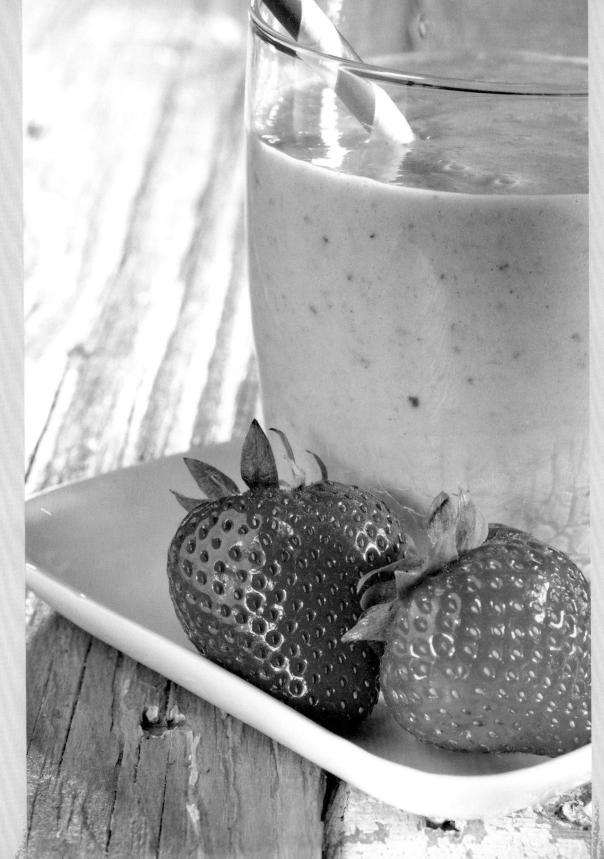

# CHAPTER 9

# Smoothies

"We stand a chance to improve
our health in a way that
has never been available
to us in the past."

—David Wolfe

Mixed-Berry Smoothie

# Banana Smoothie

*Total time:* **10 minutes** | *Serves* **2**

### INGREDIENTS:
1 cup Almond Milk (see p. 85)
2 bananas
3 seedless dates

### ACTIONS:
1. Put all ingredients in the blender.
2. Blend on high speed until the mixture reaches a smooth consistency.

### TIPS:
1. As an alternative to dates, use 1 tablespoon raw honey or maple syrup.
2. Add ⅛ teaspoon salt for more flavor.
3. Add ½ cup ice for thicker consistency.
4. Add ½ teaspoon pure vanilla extract.
5. Freeze the bananas for a thicker, cooler smoothie.

### VARIATIONS:
1. Add 1½ teaspoons of cacao powder for Chocolate Banana Smoothie.
2. Add 1½ teaspoons of cacao powder and 2 tablespoons of peanut butter for Chocolate Peanut Butter Banana Smoothie.
3. Add ½ cup berries for Banana-Berry Smoothie.
4. Freeze this smoothie for 2 hours for Banana Smoothie Ice Cream.

*Calories:* **341** | *Total Fat:* **10g**
*Carbohydrate:* **67g** | *Dietary Fiber:* **9g**
*Protein:* **6g**

### HEALTH BENEFITS:

# Green Smoothie

*Total time:* **10 minutes** | *Serves* **2**

A great way to get your greens into one good-tasting drink!

### INGREDIENTS:
1½ cup Almond Milk (see p. 85) or water
2 cups kale
2 bananas

### ACTIONS:
1. Put all ingredients in the blender.
2. Blend until the mixture reaches a smooth consistency.

### TIPS:
1. If you want it smoother, add more water.
2. Add 1 avocado, peeled.
3. Add a handful of spinach.
4. Add a handful of cilantro.
5. Add 1 cucumber.
6. Add 3 seedless dates (or 1 tablespoon of raw honey or maple syrup).
7. Add 1 tablespoon spirulina, for extra protein and vitamins.

### VARIATION:
Freeze this smoothie for 2 hours for Green Smoothie Ice Cream.

*Calories:* **230** | *Total Fat:* **10g**
*Carbohydrate:* **35g** | *Dietary Fiber:* **6g**
*Protein:* **7g**

### HEALTH BENEFITS:

# Strawberry Smoothie

*Total time:* **10 minutes** | *Serves* **1**

### INGREDIENTS:

1 cup Almond Milk (see p. 85)
   or Seed Milk (see p. 86)
1½ cups strawberries
4 seedless dates
1 cup ice

### ACTIONS:

1. Put all ingredients in the blender.
2. Blend the mixture on high speed until it reaches a smooth consistency.

### TIPS:

1. Any kind of nut milk or seed milk may be substituted for the Almond Milk.
2. Water may be substituted for the Almond Milk.
3. As an alternative to dates, use 1 tablespoon maple syrup or raw honey.
4. For additional sweetness, add more dates, maple syrup, or raw honey.
5. For more protein, add 1 tablespoon or more almond butter or Protein Powder (see p. 104).
6. Frozen strawberries can be used to make a colder smoothie.

### VARIATIONS:

1. Freeze the smoothie for 2 hours for Strawberry-Smoothie Ice Cream.
2. Add ¼ teaspoon or more pure vanilla extract for enhanced flavor and Strawberry Vanilla Smoothie.

*Calories:* **518** | *Total Fat:* **18g**
*Carbohydrate:* **91g** | *Dietary Fiber:* **14g**
*Protein:* **10g**

### HEALTH BENEFITS:

# Paradise Smoothie

*Total time:* **15 minutes** | *Serves* **3**

Best had on a sunny day on the beach!

### INGREDIENTS:

1 papaya, peeled and cut in chunks
1 pineapple, peeled and cut in chunks
9 passion fruits

### ACTIONS:

1. Peel and cut the pineapple and papaya into pieces and add to blender.
2. Scoop out the insides of the passion fruit and add to blender.
3. Blend on high speed until the mixture reaches a smooth consistency.

### TIP:

Add 1 cup of ice to the blender, if you want a cold smoothie.

### VARIATIONS:

1. Add 1 mango for Mango Paradise Smoothie.
2. Add 1 lemon for Lemon Paradise Smoothie.
3. Add 1 tablespoon coconut oil and 2 tablespoons coconut flakes for Coconut Paradise Smoothie.

*Calories:* **243** | *Total Fat:* **1g**
*Carbohydrate:* **62g** | *Dietary Fiber:* **12g**
*Protein:* **3g**

### HEALTH BENEFITS:

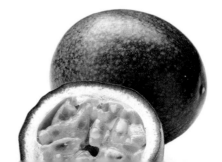

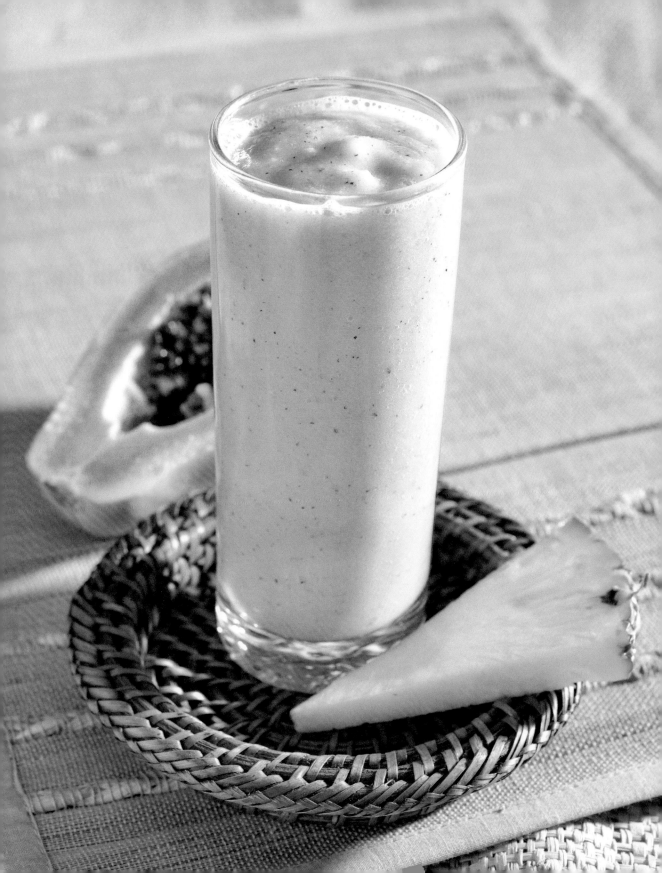

# Mixed-Berry Smoothie

*Total time:* **10 minutes**  |  *Serves* **1–2**

### INGREDIENTS:

1 cup orange juice, freshly squeezed
   (3–5 oranges) or nut/seed milk

2 cups of berries (blueberries, strawberries,
   and raspberries)

### ACTIONS:

1. Put all ingredients in the blender.
2. Blend until the mixture reaches
   a smooth consistency.

### TIPS:

1. Get closer to nature by squeezing
   the oranges by hand.
2. If the mixture is too thick for your liking,
   add more liquid—either more orange juice,
   some water, or crushed ice.
3. Add 1 teaspoon of maca powder, for
   additional health benefits.
4. Add 1 tablespoon flaxseeds or flaxseed oil
   for more benefits.
5. Substitute grapefruit juice for the
   orange juice.
6. Add the juice of 1 lemon to give your
   smoothie a kick and extra vitamin C.
7. Freeze the berries for a cooler smoothie.
8. If you freeze this smoothie it will stay good
   in the freezer for 8 weeks, a great thing to
   grab on-the-go.
9. Add honey, dates, or maple syrup if it
   is not sweet enough for you.
10. This smoothie can be made with water.

### VARIATIONS:

1. Add ⅓ cup blackberries, ⅓ cup mulberries,
   ⅓ cup goji berries, and ¼ cup water for
   Super Mixed-Berry Smoothie.
2. Add 1–2 tablespoons of almond butter for
   more protein for Nut-Berry Smoothie.
3. Freeze this smoothie for an hour for
   Mixed-Berry Smoothie Sorbet.
4. Add 2 teaspoons of cacao powder for
   Chocolate-Berry Smoothie.
5. Add 2 teaspoons cacao powder and
   2 tablespoons almond butter for
   Chocolate Nut Berry Smoothie.

*Calories:* **223**  |  *Total Fat:* **1g**
*Carbohydrate:* **53g**  |  *Dietary Fiber:* **9g**
*Protein:* **4g**

### HEALTH BENEFITS:

# Slushy

*Total time:* **10 minutes**  |  *Serves* **1**

### INGREDIENTS:

½ cup crushed ice

1 cup strawberries

2 red apples

### ACTIONS:

1. Take out the seeds from the apples.
   Put all ingredients in the blender.
2. Blend until mixture reaches a slushy
   consistency.

### TIPS:

1. Freeze your strawberries ahead of time
   so the slushy will be ice cold.
2. If you prefer a thinner consistency,
   add water.

### VARIATIONS:

1. Replace the strawberries with 1 cup of
   watermelon for Watermelon Slushy.
2. Freeze the slushy in an ice cube tray
   for Slushy Ice Cubes.

*Calories:* **235**  |  *Total Fat:* **1g**
*Carbohydrate:* **61g**  |  *Dietary Fiber:* **12g**
*Protein:* **2g**

### HEALTH BENEFITS:

# Vanilla Smoothie

*Total time:* **10 minutes** | *Serves* **1**

INGREDIENTS:

1 cup Almond Milk (see p. 85)
2 teaspoons pure vanilla extract
3 seedless dates
2 cups ice

ACTIONS:

1. Put all ingredients in the blender.
2. Blend the mixture on high speed until it reaches a smooth consistency.

TIPS:

1. Any kind of nut milk or seed milk may be substituted to make it nut free.
2. Water may be substituted for the Almond Milk.
3. As an alternative to dates, use 1 tablespoon maple syrup or honey.
4. Make it even sweeter by adding more dates, honey, or maple syrup.
5. Instead of using ice, you can use 2–3 frozen bananas.
6. Transform this smoothie by adding your favorite superfoods, such as maca powder, acai, cacao powder, coconut oil, chia seeds, ginseng, green tea, or greens powder; or any fruits, such as strawberries, blueberries, or raspberries.

*Calories:* **489** | *Total Fat:* **18g**
*Carbohydrate:* **80g** | *Dietary Fiber:* **11g**
*Protein:* **9g**

HEALTH BENEFITS:

# Chocolate Smoothie

*Total time:* **10 minutes** | *Serves* **1**

INGREDIENTS:

Make the Chocolate Shake (see p. 87)
2 cups crushed ice
3 seedless dates
1 teaspoon pure vanilla extract
1/4 teaspoon salt

ACTIONS:

1. Place all ingredients in the blender.
2. Blend until the mixture reaches a smooth consistency.

TIPS:

1. Replace the dates with 1 tablespoon raw honey or maple syrup.
2. Replace the ice with 2 frozen bananas.
3. For additional sweetness, add more dates, maple syrup, or raw honey.
4. If you prefer a darker, richer chocolate flavor, add more cacao powder.
5. Add 1 tablespoon whole chia seeds, for extra thickness and additional health benefits.

VARIATIONS:

1. Add 1 tablespoon coconut oil for Chocolate-Coconut Smoothie.
2. Add 2 teaspoons of freshly ground organic coffee beans for Chocolate-Coffee Smoothie.

*Calories:* **501** | *Total Fat:* **19g**
*Carbohydrate:* **85g** | *Dietary Fiber:* **13g**
*Protein:* **11g**

HEALTH BENEFITS:

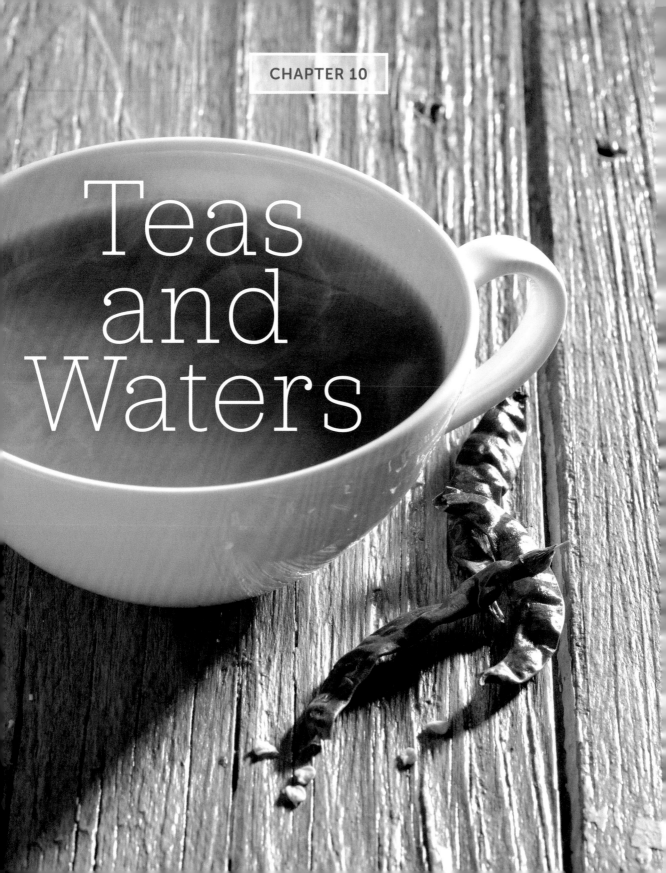

# CHAPTER 10

# Teas and Waters

> **"Surely a pretty woman never looks prettier than when making tea."**
>
> —Mary Elizabeth Braddon

# Immune-boosting Tea

*Total time:* **10 minutes** | *Serves* **1**

### INGREDIENTS:

2 cups water
1-inch piece of ginger, diced
1 garlic clove, diced
¼ teaspoon turmeric powder
A dash of cayenne pepper (it should be spicy but comfortable to drink)
1 lemon
1 tablespoon raw honey (optional)

### ACTIONS:

1. In a saucepan, bring water, ginger, garlic, and cayenne pepper to a boil. Reduce heat to medium and simmer for 7 minutes.
2. Strain as you pour into a teacup.
3. Squeeze in the juice of the lemon, add honey, and stir well.
4. Drink warm.

*Calories:* **87** | *Total Fat:* **0g**
*Carbohydrate:* **24g** | *Dietary Fiber:* **1g**
*Protein:* **1g**

### HEALTH BENEFITS:

# Weight Loss Tea

*Total time:* **10 minutes** | *Serves* **2**

### INGREDIENTS:

4 cups water
2-inch piece of ginger, diced
A dash of cayenne pepper
½ teaspoon turmeric powder
1 lemon

### ACTIONS:

1. In a saucepan, boil water, ginger, and cayenne pepper for 7 minutes.
2. Strain as you pour the liquid into teacups.
3. Squeeze in the juice of the lemon.
4. Drink warm.

### TIPS:

1. Instead of discarding the ginger, you can eat it.
2. The tea should be spicy but also comfortable for you to drink. If it's not spicy enough for you, add more cayenne pepper.

*Calories:* **14** | *Total Fat:* **0g**
*Carbohydrate:* **4g** | *Dietary Fiber:* **1g**
*Protein:* **0g**

### HEALTH BENEFITS:

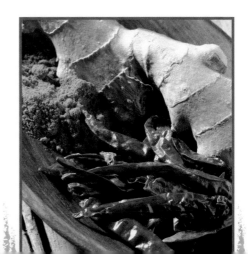

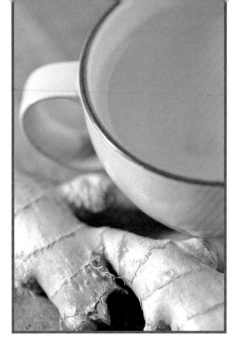

# Ginger Tea

*Total time:* **10 minutes** | *Serves* **2**

### INGREDIENTS:

4 cups water
2-inch piece of ginger, diced

### ACTIONS:

1. In a saucepan, boil water and ginger for 7 minutes.
2. Strain as you pour into teacups.
3. Drink warm.

*Calories:* **2** | *Total Fat:* **0g**
*Carbohydrate:* **0g** | *Dietary Fiber:* **0g**
*Protein:* **0g**

### HEALTH BENEFITS:

# Energy Tea

*Total time:* **10 minutes** | *Serves* **2**

### INGREDIENTS:

4 cups water
1 teaspoon fresh or dried lavender
1 teaspoon dried green tea leaves
1 teaspoon fresh or dried mint
1 teaspoon ginseng root or powder

### ACTIONS:

1. In a saucepan boil water, lavender, green tea leaves, mint, and ginseng for 5 minutes.
2. Strain as you pour into teacups.
3. Drink warm.

*Calories:* **2** | *Total Fat:* **0g**
*Carbohydrate:* **0g** | *Dietary Fiber:* **0g**
*Protein:* **0g**

### HEALTH BENEFITS:

# Relaxation Tea

*Total time:* **10 minutes** | *Serves* **2**

### INGREDIENTS:

4 cups water
2 tablespoons chamomile flowers
1 tablespoon lavender

### ACTIONS:

1. In a saucepan, boil water, chamomile, and lavender for 5 minutes.
2. Strain as you pour into teacups.
3. Drink warm.

*Calories:* **3** | *Total Fat:* **0.1g**
*Carbohydrate:* **4g** | *Dietary Fiber:* **0g**
*Protein:* **.2g**

### HEALTH BENEFITS:

# Mint Water

*Total time:* **5 minutes** | *Serves* **1**

## INGREDIENTS:

**2 cups water**
**½ cup fresh mint**

## ACTIONS:

1. Tear mint leaves from their stems and add to water.
2. Drink.

## TIP:

Place water in the fridge for 1 hour to enjoy chilled mint water.

## VARIATION:

Place the mint water in ice cube trays and freeze for 2 hours for Mint Ice Cubes.

*Calories:* **12** | *Total Fat:* **0g**
*Carbohydrate:* **1g** | *Dietary Fiber:* **0g**
*Protein:* **1g**

## HEALTH BENEFITS:

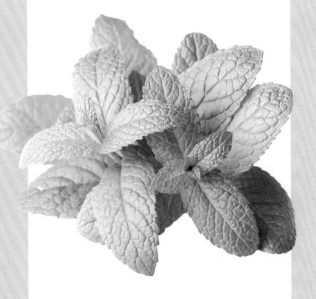

# Cucumber Water

*Total time:* **5 minute** | *Serves* **1**

## INGREDIENTS:

**2 cups water**
**1 small cucumber, thinly sliced**

## ACTIONS:

1. Place cucumber slices in water.
2. Drink.

## TIPS:

1. Place water in the fridge for 1 hour for chilled cucumber water.
2. After drinking the water, you can eat the cucumbers or pat them on your face to hydrate the skin!

## VARIATIONS:

1. Place the cucumber water in ice cube trays and freeze for 2 hours for Cucumber Ice Cubes.
2. Add a squeeze of lemon for Lemon Cucumber Water.
3. Add ½ cup raspberries for Raspberry Cucumber Water.
4. Use raspberries instead of cucumber for Raspberry Water.
5. Use strawberries instead of cucumber for Strawberry Water.

*Calories:* **2** | *Total Fat:* **0g**
*Carbohydrate:* **1g** | *Dietary Fiber:* **0g**
*Protein:* **0g**

## HEALTH BENEFITS:

# Coconut Water

*Total time:* **5 minutes** | *Serves* **1**

### INGREDIENT:

**1 fresh whole coconut**

### ACTIONS:

1. Make a hole in the coconut.
   Here is the easiest way: On one end
   of every coconut you'll see three darker
   circles together. One of the holes will
   be softer than the others. Poke through
   this hole with a screwdriver or a sharp
   kitchen utensil, like a thin knife or
   a metal chopstick.
2. Drain the coconut water into a cup,
   or place a straw in the hole and drink
   directly from the coconut!

*Calories:* **91** | *Total Fat:* **1g**
*Carbohydrate:* **18g** | *Dietary Fiber:* **5g**
*Protein:* **3g**

### HEALTH BENEFITS:

# Lemon Water

*Total time:* **5 minutes** | *Serves* **1**

### INGREDIENTS:

**2 cups water**
**1 lemon**

### ACTIONS:

1. Hand squeeze the lemon into
   the water.
2. Drink.

*Calories:* **12** | *Total Fat:* **0g**
*Carbohydrate:* **4g** | *Dietary Fiber:* **0g**
*Protein:* **0g**

### HEALTH BENEFITS:

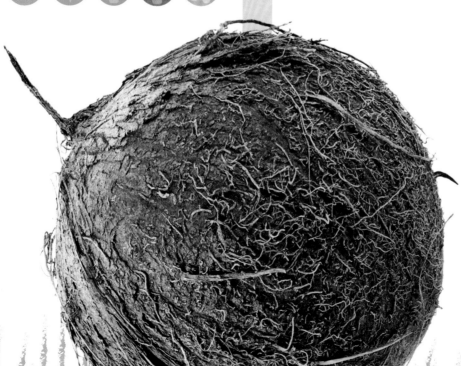

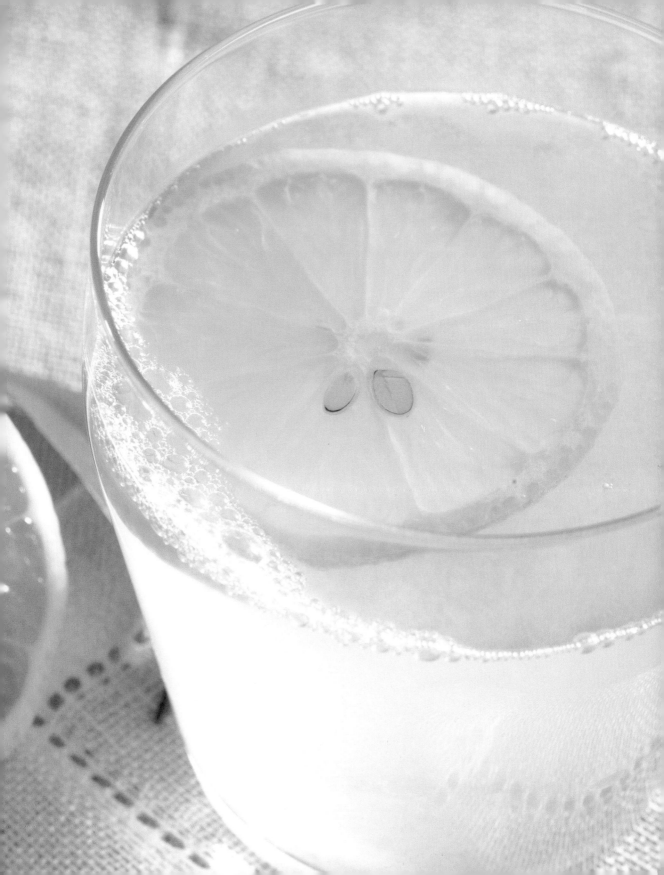

# CHAPTER 11

# Raw Vegan Main Dishes

Raw Pizza

"Following a plant-based diet dials down our insane consumption of resources like fresh water, oil, coal, and the precious rain forest. It helps to heal the environment by denying support to toxic food industries."

— Alicia Silverstone

# Breakfast Cereal

*Total time:* **15 minutes** | *Serves* **2–3**

Enjoy this delicious breakfast with a glass of Lemon Water and watch the sunrise.

### INGREDIENTS:

½ cup gluten-free rolled oats
½ cup raw macadamia nuts
½ cup blueberries
½ cup almond meal
1 apple, cored
1 teaspoon cinnamon (or more, to taste)
¼ cup raw walnuts
1 teaspoon raw honey or maple syrup
1–2 cups Almond Milk (see p. 85)
Additional honey or maple syrup (optional)

### ACTIONS:

1. In a bowl, toss together the rolled oats, macadamia nuts, blueberries, and almond meal. Set aside.
2. In a food processor, blend the apple, cinnamon, walnuts, and honey (or maple syrup) until the mixture reaches a crumbled consistency. If the mixture does not begin sticking together in clumps, add a bit more honey.
3. Take mixture from the food processor and roll into loose balls about 1 inch in diameter. Add these to the bowl with the rolled oats mixture to complete your breakfast cereal.
4. Pour Almond Milk over your cereal.
5. Add additional honey or maple syrup for sweetness, to taste.

### TIPS:

1. Add any raw nuts and fruits of your choice.
2. Sprinkle 1 tablespoon of psyllium husks over the cereal for added health benefits.
3. Sprinkle 1 tablespoon of flaxseeds over cereal for added health benefits.

*Calories:* **502** | *Total Fat:* **37g**
*Carbohydrate:* **40g** | *Dietary Fiber:* **10g**
*Protein:* **11g**

### HEALTH BENEFITS:

# Protein Powder

*Total time:* **5 minutes** | *Serves* **1**

### INGREDIENTS:
**½ cup of pumpkin seeds**

### ACTIONS:
In a high-speed blender, mix the pumpkin seeds until they're chopped fine with no chunks at all.

### TIPS:
1. Mix the pumpkin seed meal with 2 cups of water, nut milk or Seed Milk for a protein drink, or add it to smoothies and juices for extra protein.
2. Make 3 ½ cups of pumpkin seed meal and store in a jar and keep in the fridge or at room temperature for one week's supply.
3. Sprinkle it on cereals or salads.

### VARIATIONS:
1. Use hemp seeds for Hemp Seed Protein Powder (30g protein per ½ cup powder).
2. Use raw peanuts for Peanut Protein Powder (19g protein per ½ cup powder).
3. Use almonds for Almond Protein Powder (16g protein per ½ cup powder).
4. Use uncooked quinoa for Quinoa Protein Powder (12g protein per ½ cup powder).
5. Use uncooked brown rice for Brown Rice Protein Powder (7.5g protein per ½ cup powder).

*Calories:* **374** | *Total Fat:* **32g**
*Carbohydrate:* **13g** | *Dietary Fiber:* **3g**
*Protein:* **17g**

### HEALTH BENEFITS:

# Three-ingredient Chia Seed Cereal

*Total time:* **10 minutes** | *Serves* **1**

### INGREDIENTS:
**3 tablespoons chia seeds**
**½ cup water, nut milk, or Seed Milk (see p. 86)**
**Your choice of chopped fruit: one apple, banana, peach, pear, nectarine, or ½ cup berries**

### ACTIONS:
1. Place the chia seeds and liquid into a cereal bowl. Soak for 5 minutes.
2. Add the fruit and eat!

### TIP:
Add 1 teaspoon of raw honey, maple syrup, or chopped dates if you want it sweeter.

### VARIATIONS:
1. Add 1 tablespoon of hemp seeds for Chia Hemp Seed Cereal.
2. Add 1 tablespoon of oats for Oatmeal Chia Seed Cereal.

*Calories:* **87** | *Total Fat:* **8g**
*Carbohydrate:* **9g** | *Dietary Fiber:* **8g**
*Protein:* **5g**

### HEALTH BENEFITS:

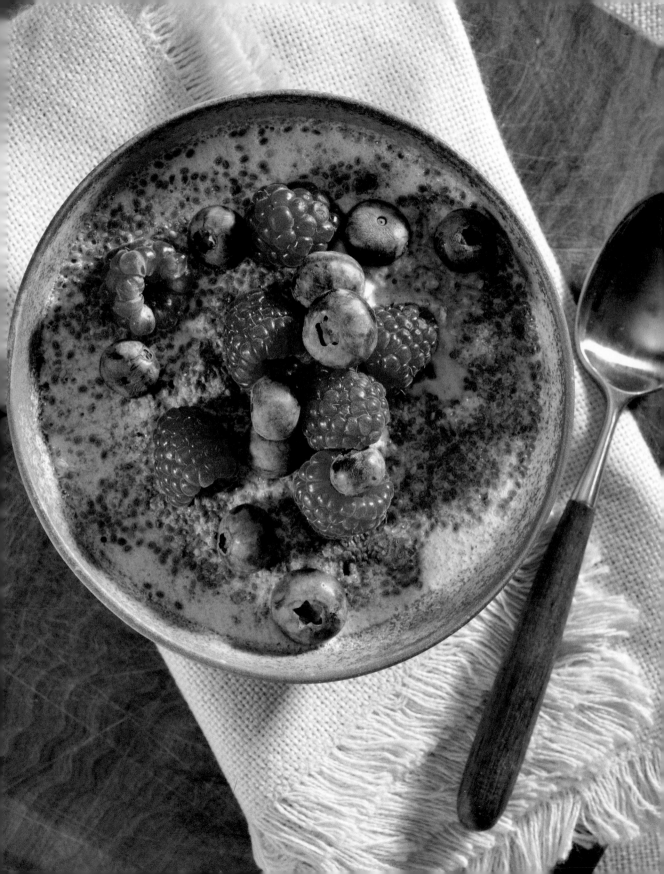

# Green Salad

*Total time:* **25 minutes** | *Serves* **4**

INGREDIENTS:

1 head any kind of lettuce, torn into
    small pieces
1 bunch kale including the stems and ribs,
    torn into small pieces
10 asparagus stalks, halved (don't
    include the bottom inch or so,
    which can be tough)
1 avocado, cut into cubes or slices
1 cucumber, chopped into cubes
1 garlic clove, diced
1-inch piece of ginger, diced
1 purple onion, chopped in thin slices
1 cup alfalfa sprouts
1 green apple, chopped into thin slices
1 celery stalk, chopped into cubes
¼ cup extra-virgin olive oil (to drizzle)
Juice of 1 lemon (to drizzle)

ACTIONS:

1. Combine all the ingredients, except oil
    and lemon juice, in a bowl and toss.
2. Drizzle with olive oil and lemon juice.

TIP:

Add 1 large radish, finely sliced, for extra
flavor and nutrients.

VARIATIONS:

1. 1 green chili, chopped into small pieces
    for Spicy Green Salad.
2. ½ cup of walnuts, to make it crunchy
    for Nutty Green Salad.
3. 3 tablespoons raw honey or maple syrup
    for Sweet Green Salad.
4. Add 2 bell peppers (any color), chopped in
    small pieces, for Crunchy Green Salad.
5. Add ¾ cup of any type of beans, for
    Bean Green Salad.

*Calories:* **287** | *Total Fat:* **20g**
*Carbohydrate:* **28g** | *Dietary Fiber:* **8g**
*Protein:* **7g**

HEALTH BENEFITS:

# Four-ingredient Green Salad

*Total time:* **10 minutes** | *Serves* **1**

INGREDIENTS:

1 avocado
1 cup fresh parsley leaves
1 cup fresh cilantro leaves
1 lemon

ACTIONS:

1. Chop the avocado into cubes.
2. Place the avocado, parsley, and cilantro in
    a bowl. Squeeze the lemon over the salad.

TIPS:

1. Add salt and pepper to taste.
2. Include the stems from the parsley and
    cilantro for added nutrients.

VARIATION:

Add 1 chopped cucumber for Five-ingredient
Green Salad.

*Calories:* **332** | *Total Fat:* **27g**
*Carbohydrate:* **23g** | *Dietary Fiber:* **16g**
*Protein:* **7g**

HEALTH BENEFITS:

# Superfood Kale Salad

*Total time:* **10 minutes**
*Serves* **3**

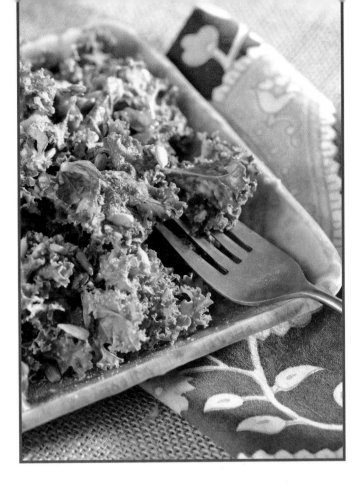

## INGREDIENTS:

1 bunch kale, center ribs and stems removed (save stems and ribs for juicing or eating later)
1 avocado
1 tablespoon apple cider vinegar
1½ tablespoons flaxseed oil
¾ teaspoon salt
4 tablespoons nutritional yeast
5 tablespoons sunflower seeds

## ACTIONS:

1. Tear the kale leaves into small pieces and place in large bowl.
2. Massage the avocado into the pieces of kale with your fingers, covering the kale with avocado.
3. Add remaining ingredients to the bowl and stir, or continue to massage the mixture with your fingers, until everything is well combined.

## TIPS:

1. Add more of any of the ingredients to taste.
2. Increase the amount of nutritional yeast if you would like the salad to have a cheesy flavor.
3. Add pumpkin seeds for more protein.

## VARIATIONS:

1. Roll up salad in a brown rice wrap for portable Kale Wraps.
2. Add 2 teaspoons of garlic powder for Garlic Kale Salad.

*Calories:* **426** | *Total Fat:* **24g**
*Carbohydrate:* **35g** | *Dietary Fiber:* **17g**
*Protein:* **29g**

## HEALTH BENEFITS:

PROTEIN | WEIGHT LOSS | AO | ANTI-INFLAM. | DH

# Cashew Cheese

*Total time:* **10 minutes**  |  *Makes* **1 cup, serves 4**

## INGREDIENTS:

2 cups cashews

2 tablespoons nutritional yeast

Juice of 1 small lemon (no more
than ¼ cup)

½ teaspoon salt

½ cup water (more for a softer cheese)

## ACTIONS:

1. Put all ingredients in your food processor.
2. Blend mixture until smooth.

## TIPS:

1. Soak the cashews for 4 hours for
   a smoother, creamier cheese.
2. For a nut free version, instead of cashews,
   use hemp seeds, pumpkin seeds, or
   sunflower seeds.
3. This recipe also works with almonds,
   macadamia, walnuts, and brazil nuts.
4. For a cheesier flavor, add more nutritional
   yeast, to taste. You can also make this
   recipe without nutritional yeast.
5. Serve on Raw Tacos (see p. 113) or
   Raw Pizza (see p. 112), or in Raw Lasagna
   (see p. 110) or on lettuce for Lettuce Wraps.
6. Add a dash of cayenne pepper or chili
   flakes for spice.
7. Add 1 teaspoon thyme for more flavor.

## VARIATIONS:

1. To make Raw Parmesan Cheese, add an
   extra 3 tablespoons nutritional yeast to
   the mixture and spread the mixture
   ¼-inch thick on a dehydrator tray. Place
   in a food dehydrator for 12 hours. It will
   crumble easily when you're ready to use it.
2. Add one garlic clove or more for
   Garlic Cashew Cheese.
3. Add 1 cup fresh basil leaves for
   Pesto Cashew Cheese.

*Calories:* **486**  |  *Total Fat:* **37g**
*Carbohydrate:* **30g**  |  *Dietary Fiber:* **4g**
*Protein:* **17g**

## HEALTH BENEFITS:

# Guacamole

*Total time:* **5 minutes**  |  *Serves* **1**

## INGREDIENTS:

1 avocado

¼ teaspoon salt

¼ teaspoon black pepper

Juice of ½ lemon

## ACTIONS:

1. Mash the avocado in a bowl with a fork.
2. Blend in the other ingredients.

## TIPS:

1. Eat with carrot sticks.
2. Eat with cucumber sticks.
3. Add ½ small purple onion, diced.
4. Add ½ small pepper (bell) any color, diced.

*Calories:* **234**  |  *Total Fat:* **21g**
*Carbohydrate:* **14g**  |  *Dietary Fiber:* **9g**
*Protein:* **3g**

## HEALTH BENEFITS:

# Walnut Meat Mixture

*Total time:* **10 minutes** | *Serves* **4–6**

## INGREDIENTS:

1½ cups walnuts
1 cup sundried tomatoes
2 tablespoons extra-virgin olive oil
1 tablespoon fresh sage
1 teaspoon fennel seeds
1 teaspoon fresh thyme
1 teaspoon fresh rosemary
1 teaspoon fresh oregano
1 pinch black pepper
1 pinch cayenne pepper
1 pinch salt

## ACTION:

Add all ingredients to your blender and mix for 5 minutes or until well combined.

## TIPS:

1. If you do not have a blender, you can make this recipe using a mortar and pestle. Crush the walnuts first. Dice the sundried tomatoes and mix everything together in a bowl until it is moist enough to stick together.
2. This recipe can be used as the meat for Raw Burgers, Raw Tacos, Raw Pizza, Zucchini Pasta and Walnut Meat Balls, and Raw Lasagna.
3. For a nut-free version, use pumpkin or sunflower seeds instead of walnuts.
4. If you cannot get fresh herbs, use dried.

*Calories:* **274** | *Total Fat:* **25g**
*Carbohydrate:* **10g** | *Dietary Fiber:* **4g**
*Protein:* **6g**

## HEALTH BENEFITS:

# Raw Burgers

*Total time:* **40 minutes** | *Makes* **4**

## INGREDIENTS:

1 Walnut Meat Mixture
1 Cashew Cheese (see p. 108)
4 large collard/kale leaves or
    4 Gluten-free Rolls (see p. 133)
Topping of your choice, such as
    avocado, ketchup, mustard, lettuce

## ACTIONS:

1. Form Walnut Meat Mixture into 4 patties.
2. Place the patties on collard/kale leaves or rolls.
3. Top your burger with Cashew Cheese and whatever else you like.

## TIP:

Serve with French Fries (see p. 119) for a hybrid—part raw/part cooked—meal!

*Calories:* **399** | *Total Fat:* **39g**
*Carbohydrate:* **17g** | *Dietary Fiber:* **8g**
*Protein:* **19g**

## HEALTH BENEFITS:

# Raw Lasagna

*Total time:* **40 minutes** | *Makes* **12 slices,** **serves 12**

### INGREDIENTS:

1 Walnut Meat Mixture (see p. 109)
1 Cashew Cheese (see p. 108)
2 large zucchinis
1 cup fresh spinach
1 cup fresh basil
1 tablespoon dried oregano
   for sprinkling
2 tablespoons extra-virgin olive oil

### ACTIONS:

1. Peel and slice the zucchini into thin strips, with a vegetable peeler. Place the first layer of zucchini in a deep lasagna dish (8 x 11½ x 2-inch baking dish), which holds 2 quarts. Layer zucchini so that strips are just overlapping each other. You could also build the lasagna directly on plates if you will be eating it immediately. Sprinkle ½ tablespoon of oregano over the zucchini strips.
2. Add a layer of the Walnut Meat Mixture. Use half of it keeping in mind you will create another layer later.
3. Spread ½ cup Cashew Cheese over Walnut Meat Mixture.
4. Place half cup each of spinach and basil leaves over Cashew Cheese.
5. Add another layer of zucchini strips (keep in mind you will need one more layer for top of lasagna).
6. Repeat the layering of Walnut Meat Mixture, Cashew Cheese, basil, and spinach.
7. Add the last layer of zucchini strips and sprinkle with the remaining ½ tablespoon oregano. Finish with a drizzle of extra-virgin olive oil.
8. It is now ready to eat, but if you allow it to set in the refrigerator overnight it will be easier to slice.

### TIPS:

1. If you want to add more layers, add the pesto sauce from the Zucchini Pasta with Pesto recipe and the Raw Tomato Sauce.
2. This keeps well in the fridge for 4–5 days.
3. If you want a spicy lasagna, sprinkle cayenne pepper on one of the layers.

*Calories:* **307** | *Total Fat:* **25g**
*Carbohydrate:* **17g** | *Dietary Fiber:* **4g**
*Protein:* **9g**

### HEALTH BENEFITS:

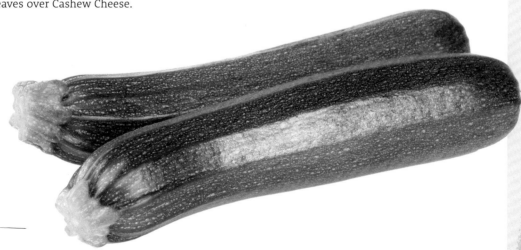

# Raw Crackers

*Total time:* **20 minutes to assemble,**
**12 hours to set in refrigerator,**
**15–20 hours to dehydrate** | *Serves* **20**

## INGREDIENTS:

3 cups ground flaxseeds
1 cup sunflower seeds
2 tablespoons minced onion
   (or 3 tablespoons onion powder)
2 tablespoons sesame seeds
1 tablespoon minced garlic
   (or 2 tablespoons garlic powder)
2 teaspoons cumin powder
1 teaspoon chili powder
1 teaspoon salt
1 teaspoon cayenne pepper
½ teaspoon turmeric
½ cup water

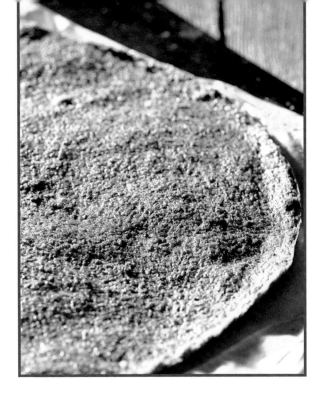

## ACTIONS:

1. Put all the dry ingredients in the bowl of a food processor and blend until a fine, flourlike consistency is achieved.
2. Add water and mix until a batter forms. Cover, and allow the batter to set in fridge for 12 hours.
3. Then spread a ⅛-inch layer of batter on non-stick dehydrator sheets and dehydrate at 100°F for 15–20 hours. For an oven alternative see tips. Cut into 20 pieces. Store in airtight container at room temperature or in the fridge. Can last up to 8 weeks.

## TIPS:

1. For an oven alternative to the dehydrator, place a layer of batter on non-stick baking paper or a baking sheet lightly greased with coconut oil and place in the oven at 180°F for 2–4 hours. The batter becomes a base when it is crisp and dry; check frequently. Cut into cracker squares.
2. Serve these crackers with Hummus (see p. 120), Tahini (see p. 120), Pesto (see p. 114), and/or Cashew Cheese (see p. 108).
3. This can be the base of the Raw Pizza (see p. 112) as well as Raw Tacos (see p. 113).

*Calories:* **277** | *Total Fat:* **22g**
*Carbohydrate:* **14g** | *Dietary Fiber:* **11g**
*Protein:* **10g**

## HEALTH BENEFITS:

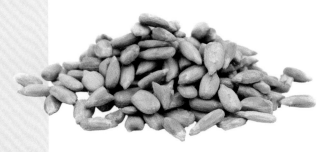

# Raw Pizza

*Total time:* **35 minutes to assemble**

*Makes* **1 large pizza, serves 10–12**

## INGREDIENTS:

*For the base*

**Use the Raw Crackers recipe (p. 111),
   formed into a 12 x 12-inch square**

*For the topping*

**Raw Tomato Sauce (p. 113)**

**Cashew Cheese (p. 108)**

**Pesto (p. 114)**

**Walnut Meat Mixture (p. 109)**

## ACTION:

Place your toppings on the base in this order:
Tomato Sauce, Cashew Cheese, Pesto Sauce,
and Walnut Meat Mixture.

## VARIATION:

For faster prep, use the Quick Bread recipe
(see p. 132) as a base. Note that this variation
is not 100 percent raw, but a Hybrid Pizza.

*Calories:* **458** | *Total Fat:* **37g**
*Carbohydrate:* **27g** | *Dietary Fiber:* **9g**
*Protein:* **15g**

## HEALTH BENEFITS:

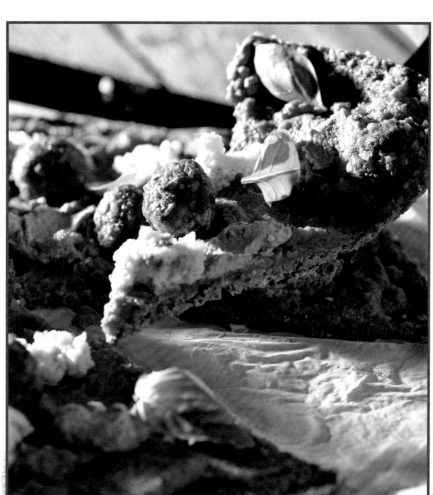

# Raw Tomato Sauce

*Total time:* **10 minutes, plus 30 minutes soaking time** | *Serves* **4**

## INGREDIENTS:

2 large tomatoes
1 cup sundried tomatoes, soaked
 for 30 minutes
1 garlic clove
¼ red or yellow onion
1 tablespoon extra-virgin olive oil
¼ teaspoon black pepper
¼ teaspoon chili flakes or
 cayenne pepper
1 tablespoon fresh basil, or
 ½ tablespoon dried basil
½ teaspoon dried thyme
½ teaspoon dried parsley
½ teaspoon dried oregano

## ACTION:

Add all ingredients to the blender and mix for one minute or until well combined.

## TIP.

Serve this sauce with the Zucchini Pasta and Walnut Meat Balls (see p. 115), Raw Tacos (see p. 113), Raw Pizza (see p. 112), and as an extra layer on the Raw Lasagna (see p. 110).

*Calories:* **70** | *Total Fat:* **3g**
*Carbohydrate:* **10g** | *Dietary Fiber:* **3g**
*Protein:* **2g**

## HEALTH BENEFITS:

# Raw Tacos

*Total time:* **20 minutes** | *Serves* **4**

## INGREDIENTS:

1 head lettuce (or collard greens)
1 Walnut Meat Mixture (see p. 109)

## ACTIONS:

1. Lay out individual lettuce leaves
 (or collard greens) on plates.
2. Put a modest portion of walnut meat
 filling into each of the lettuce leaves.
3. Add toppings of your choice
 (see Tips below).
4. Fold lettuce to form the completed
 tacos.

## TIPS:

1. Serve with toppings of chopped
 avocado, spring onions, grated carrot,
 Cashew Cheese (see p. 108), and
 Vegan Sour Cream (see p. 151) for
 a full taco experience.
2. If you have nut allergies, substitute
 sunflower seeds or hemp seeds for
 the walnuts.

## VARIATION:

You can also make hard taco shells by using the base in the Raw Crackers recipe (see p. 111). Divide the batter into eighths. After 7 hours, remove batter from dehydrator and cut out 8 circles, folding them into shells. Return shells to dehydrator, and continue to dehydrate for another 10–12 hours until crisp. Fill with your toppings for Raw Crispy Shell Tacos.

*Calories:* **356** | *Total Fat:* **32g**
*Carbohydrate:* **16g** | *Dietary Fiber:* **6g**
*Protein:* **9g**

## HEALTH BENEFITS:

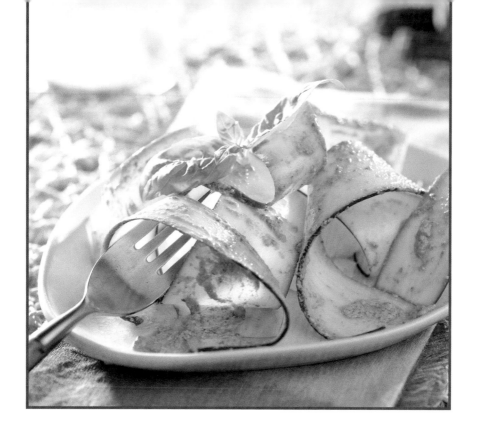

# Zucchini Pasta
# with Pesto

*Total time:* **20 minutes** | *Serves* **4**

### INGREDIENTS:

4 large zucchinis
1 cup fresh basil
Juice of 1 lemon
4 garlic cloves
½ teaspoon salt
½ cup spinach
2 cups raw walnuts
½ cup extra-virgin olive oil
   (or more for smoother mixture)

### ACTIONS:

1. Make thin strips of zucchini using
   a vegetable peeler or pasta machine.
   Set aside.
2. Put the other ingredients together in a
   blender and blend until mixture reaches
   desired consistency. Set aside.

3. Distribute the zucchini evenly among
   four serving dishes.
4. Pour the sauce over the pasta.

### TIPS:

1. Top the dish with Cashew Cheese
   (see p. 108).
2. Use pumpkin seeds instead of walnuts
   for a nut-free version.

*Calories:* **627** | *Total Fat:* **60g**
*Carbohydrate:* **20g** | *Dietary Fiber:* **7g**
*Protein:* **12g**

### HEALTH BENEFITS:

# Thai Wraps

*Total time:* **20 minutes** | *Serves* **4**

INGREDIENTS:

*Sauce*
1 tablespoon garlic, minced
1 tablespoon ginger, minced
2 teaspoons apple cider vinegar
1 carrot, grated
Juice of 2 oranges
¼ cup green onion, diced

*Filling*
1 cup cabbage, diced (¼ of
   a whole cabbage)
1 avocado
1 mango
4 large leaves of lettuce, kale,
   or collard greens (¼ head)
½ cup fresh mint
½ cup fresh cilantro
½ cup sprouts

ACTIONS:

1. In a bowl, make the sauce by adding
   the garlic, ginger, apple cider vinegar,
   carrot, orange juice, and green onion.
   Mix well and let sit.
2. Cut the avocado and mango into slices.
3. Lay out a large lettuce leaf and layer
   it with the avocado and mango slices,
   some mint, cilantro, sprouts, and
   cabbage. Repeat for four of them.
4. Pour some sauce over the wrap
   to taste.

*Calories:* **135** | *Total Fat:* **6g**
*Carbohydrate:* **22g** | *Dietary Fiber:* **5g**
*Protein:* **3g**

HEALTH BENEFITS:

# Zucchini Pasta and Walnut Meat Balls

*Total time:* **40 minutes** | *Serves* **4**

INGREDIENTS:

4 zucchinis
1 Raw Tomato Sauce (p. 113)
1 Walnut Meat Mixture (p. 109)
1 Cashew Cheese (p. 108)
Sprinkle of oregano

ACTIONS:

1. Use a pasta spiral or a vegetable peeler
   to make pasta strips out of the zucchini.
   Put one zucchini's worth of pasta into
   each of four bowls and set aside.
2. Roll the Walnut Meat Mixture into
   balls ½-inch in size. Place them on the
   zucchini pasta.
3. Pour the Raw Tomato Sauce evenly
   over each bowl.
4. Top with Cashew Cheese and sprinkle
   with oregano.

TIPS:

1. Serve with fresh cilantro or parsley.
2. For a simpler dish, you can make this
   without the Tomato Sauce and Cashew
   Cheese. Just the zucchini pasta and walnut
   meat balls alone make a tasty meal.

VARIATION:

Add ¼ teaspoon cayenne pepper
(or more to taste) to the Walnut Meat
Mixture for Zucchini Pasta and Spicy
Walnut Meat Balls.

*Calories:* **145** | *Total Fat:* **16g**
*Carbohydrate:* **13g** | *Dietary Fiber:* **6g**
*Protein:* **11g**

HEALTH BENEFITS:

# CHAPTER 12

# Cooked Vegan Main Dishes

Coconut Basil Sweet Potato Fries

> **"Cooking is, without a doubt, one of the most important skills a person can ever learn. Once someone has that knowledge, that's it, they're set for life."**
>
> — Jamie Oliver

# Coconut Bacon

*Total time:* **30 minutes** | *Makes* **3 ¹/₂ cups**

Stored in an airtight container at room temperature, it will keep for seven days.

### INGREDIENTS:

**3 cups coconut flakes**
**³/₄ cup apple cider vinegar**
**¹/₄ cup maple syrup**
**1 tablespoon salt**
**1 tablespoon paprika**
**2 teaspoons garlic powder**
**1 teaspoon onion salt**
**¹/₂ teaspoon dried cilantro**
**¹/₂ teaspoon dried parsley**

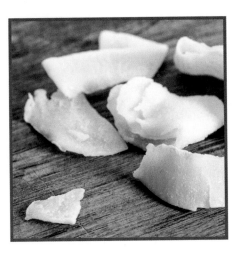

### ACTIONS:

1. Preheat oven to 250°F.
2. In a bowl, mix all ingredients, except coconut flakes, with a spoon until well combined.
3. Add the coconut flakes and stir around until the sauce has covered all of them.
4. Soak coconut flakes for 10 minutes.
5. Place coconut flakes on baking sheet or other oven-proof dish so flakes are spread out evenly and not overlapping each other. Bake for 5–12 minutes, or until the coconut flakes are crispy and golden brown.

### TIP:

Serve on salads, Raw Tacos (see p. 113), Raw Pizza (see p. 112), or wraps, with eggs or with Omelet (see p. 141).

*Calories:* **247** | *Total Fat:* **20g**
*Carbohydrate:* **18g** | *Dietary Fiber:* **5g**
*Protein:* **2g**

### HEALTH BENEFITS:

# Bean Burgers

*Total time:* **20 minutes** | *Makes* **4 burgers**

## INGREDIENTS:

One 15-ounce can of organic beans (butter
beans, kidney beans, or black beans
work best). Or you can soak dry beans
overnight, then boil them for an hour or
until soft, instead of using canned.

½ cup almond meal (blended almond)

1 small yellow onion, chopped

¼ cup nutritional yeast

½ teaspoon cumin

¼ teaspoon garlic powder

¼ teaspoon fennel

¼ teaspoon thyme

¼ teaspoon sage

¼ teaspoon salt

¼ teaspoon black pepper

⅛ teaspoon cayenne pepper

1 Flax Egg Alternative (see p. 150)

2 tablespoons extra-virgin coconut oil

## ACTIONS:

1. Drain the beans. In a bowl, mash the beans
   and mix in remaining ingredients, except
   for the oil. Taste and add more spices or
   salt to your liking. Divide into 4 equal parts
   and shape into patties.

2. Heat the oil in a large pan over medium
   heat. Fry the patties until golden, about
   4–5 minutes on each side.

3. Serve on Gluten-free Rolls (see p. 133),
   Quick Bread (see p. 132), kale, collard
   greens, or lettuce. The burgers taste great
   with herbs like fresh parsley, cilantro,
   and basil.

## TIPS:

1. Non-vegans can use one egg in this recipe
   instead of Flax Egg Alternative.

2. This meal goes great with Ketchup
   (see p. 150) and French Fries (see p. 119)!

3. You can make this recipe without
   nutritional yeast for a less cheesy flavor.
   Just replace the nutritional yeast with more
   almond meal.

4. For a nut-free version of this recipe, replace
   the almond meal with pumpkin seed,
   sunflower seed, or hemp seed meal.

## VARIATIONS:

1. Add extra cayenne pepper for Spicy
   Bean Burgers.

2. Roll the mixture into 10 balls for Bean Balls.
   Serve on brown rice pasta, Pasta Primavera,
   or Zucchini Pasta.

3. Use chickpeas instead of beans for
   Chickpea Burgers.

4. Use lentils instead of beans for Lentil
   Burgers.

*Calories:* **248** | *Total Fat:* **12g**
*Carbohydrate:* **27g** | *Dietary Fiber:* **11g**
*Protein:* **13g**

## HEALTH BENEFITS:

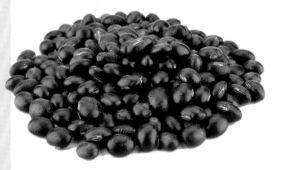

# French Fries

*Total time:* **15 minutes** | *Serves* **2**

## INGREDIENTS:

**2 large potatoes, peeled**
**½ cup extra-virgin coconut oil**
**Salt, for seasoning**

## ACTIONS:

1. Slice the potatoes into the shape of French fries.
2. In a large frying pan, heat oil over medium-high heat.
3. When oil is hot and starting to sizzle, add the potatoes.
4. Cook the fries on one side until golden brown, then flip. Fries should be crispy on the outside and soft on the inside.
5. Remove when done and drain on paper towels.

## TIP:

Serve with Ketchup (see p. 150).

## VARIATIONS:

1. Replace the white potatoes with sweet potatoes for Sweet Potato Fries.
2. Sprinkle ½ teaspoon cayenne pepper over the fries for Spicy French Fries.
3. Sprinkle 2 tablespoons nutritional yeast over the fries for Cheese Fries.
4. Sprinkle 1 tablespoon chipotle spice for Chipotle Fries.
5. Bake in oven instead of frying with oil for Baked French Fries.

*Calories:* **754** | *Total Fat:* **55g**
*Carbohydrate:* **68g** | *Dietary Fiber:* **8g**
*Protein:* **7g**

## HEALTH BENEFITS:

# Cauliflower Popcorn

*Total time:* **25 minutes** | *Serves* **4**

## INGREDIENTS:

**3 tablespoons extra-virgin olive oil**
**¼ cup nutritional yeast**
**¾ teaspoon salt**
**1 head of cauliflower, chopped into bite size pieces**

## ACTIONS:

1. Preheat oven to 325°F.
2. In a large bowl mix the olive oil, nutritional yeast, and salt until well combined.
3. Add the cauliflower pieces to bowl and toss until pieces are well coated.
4. Place the cauliflower on a baking sheet and bake for 20 minutes until golden brown and crispy.

## TIP:

Add 1 tablespoon sesame seeds for extra flavor.

## VARIATION:

If you want a cleaner dish, roast the cauliflower without any other ingredients for Plain Roasted Cauliflower, deliciously simple!

*Calories:* **135** | *Total Fat:* **4.5g**
*Carbohydrate:* **11g** | *Dietary Fiber:* **5g**
*Protein:* **9g**

## HEALTH BENEFITS:

# Tahini

*Total time:* **10 minutes** | *Serves* **4–6**

### INGREDIENTS:

½ cup of water
8 tablespoons sesame seeds
4 teaspoons sesame oil
¾ teaspoon salt

### ACTION:

Place all ingredients in the bowl of a food processor and blend until smooth.

### TIPS:

1. Use this in the Hummus recipe (below).
2. Goes great with Quick Bread (p. 132) and Raw Tacos (see p. 113).
3. Tahini makes a great salad dressing!
4. Add this to Guacamole (see p. 108).

*Calories:* **143** | *Total Fat:* **13g**
*Carbohydrate:* **4g** | *Dietary Fiber:* **2g**
*Protein:* **3g**

### HEALTH BENEFITS:

# Hummus

*Total time:* **10 minutes** | *Serves* **4–6**

### INGREDIENTS:

2 cups organic dried chickpeas (or one 14-ounce can)
¼ cup chickpea water, either from the water remaining after boiling the chickpeas or from the can
1 tablespoon extra-virgin olive oil
3 garlic cloves
1 tablespoon lemon juice
3 tablespoons Tahini (above)
1 teaspoon salt

### ACTIONS:

1. If you are using dried chickpeas, soak them overnight in the fridge, unless the temperature is cooler; then they can be left on the counter. If they are left in a hot area they can mold. The next day, add 2 teaspoons of baking soda to a pot and stir-fry the chickpeas with baking soda for 5 minutes. Add 4 cups of water and bring to a boil. Reduce heat and simmer uncovered for 15–40 minutes until chickpeas are soft.
2. Place the cooked chickpeas and all other ingredients in a food processor and blend until smooth.

### TIPS:

1. Serve with carrot and cucumber sticks.
2. Goes great with Quick Bread (p. 132) and Raw Crackers (p. 111).
3. As an alternative to chickpeas use almonds, pumpkin seeds, sunflower seeds, or hemp seeds.

### VARIATION:

Hummus makes a great salad dressing. It can be thinned by mixing in the juice of a lemon and some olive oil. Or leave it as is and massage it into kale or lettuce for a thicker, creamier Hummus Dressing.

*Calories:* **372** | *Total Fat:* **12g**
*Carbohydrate:* **51g** | *Dietary Fiber:* **15g**
*Protein:* **17g**

### HEALTH BENEFITS:

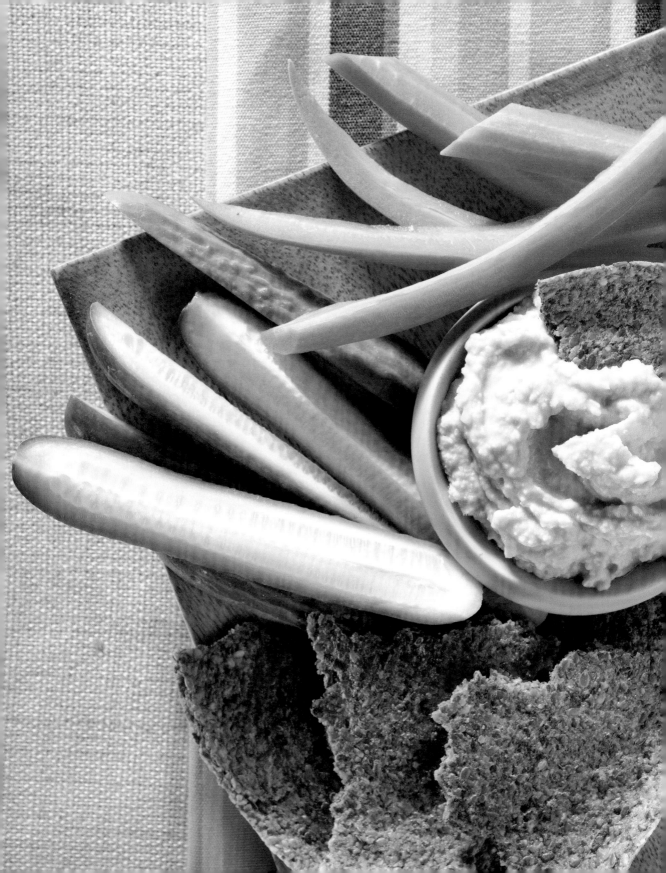

# Mac 'n' Cheese

*Total time:* **20 minutes** | *Serves* **3**

### INGREDIENTS:

3 ¼ cups water
2 cups uncooked brown rice or quinoa pasta
3 tablespoons of nutritional yeast
1 teaspoon salt

### ACTIONS:

1. In a pot, add the brown rice pasta to water.
   Bring it to a boil over high heat. Stir the
   pasta and reduce the heat to medium-low.
   Keep stirring until the pasta is soft,
   10–20 minutes. As it cooks, the pasta
   will soak up the water and begin to take
   on a creamy appearance.
   *Note:* Usually when we cook pasta, there
   is much more water in the pot and then
   the pasta is drained. But for this dish to
   succeed and achieve a natural creaminess,
   we need the pasta to soak up the water.
   The residual liquid in the pot will become
   the base for the creamy sauce, so do not
   drain it.
2. Add the nutritional yeast and the salt to the
   pot of pasta and stir until well combined
   with the water to form the sauce.

### TIPS:

1. Add 1–2 teaspoons thyme for flavor.
2. Add 1 tablespoon coconut oil, for extra
   smoothness and additional health benefits.
3. Use extra nutritional yeast if you like
   a cheesier taste, or if needed to soak up
   some liquid.

### VARIATIONS:

1. Add 1 tablespoon of pepper and stir in at
   the end for Peppery Mac 'n' Cheese.
2. Replace brown rice pasta with brown rice
   for Risotto. Then add mushrooms, onion,
   and tomatoes to flavor your Risotto.

*Calories:* **473** | *Total Fat:* **5g**
*Carbohydrate:* **92g** | *Dietary Fiber:* **5g**
*Protein:* **15g**

### HEALTH BENEFITS:

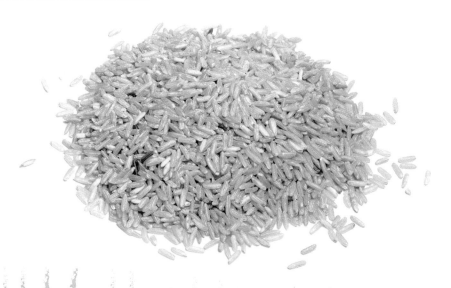

# Pasta Primavera

*Total time:* **30 minutes** | *Serves* **4**

INGREDIENTS:

2 cups uncooked brown rice or
   quinoa pasta
½ cup extra-virgin coconut oil
1 yellow onion, chopped
2 garlic cloves, diced
½ head broccoli including the stems (2–3
   cups), chopped into bite-sized pieces
1 cup fresh or frozen peas
Cracked black pepper and salt, to taste

ACTIONS:

1. Place pasta in a large pot and cover
   with 5 cups water. Bring to a boil over
   high heat. Stir pasta and reduce heat to
   medium-low. Cook 10–15 minutes. until
   tender, but not mushy.
2. While pasta cooks, heat oil in a frying
   pan over medium heat and add onion
   and garlic. Fry, stirring frequently, until
   golden brown.
3. Add broccoli to the frying pan.
   Continue cooking, stirring frequently,
   until broccoli is just tender.
4. Add cooked pasta to the vegetables and
   toss to combine. Immediately add the
   peas and toss again for a few minutes
   until flavors and oils are combined.
5. Add salt and pepper to taste.

TIP:

Add other vegetables!

VARIATION:

Add 1 teaspoon cayenne pepper for
Spicy Pasta Primavera.

*Calories:* **307** | *Total Fat:* **30g**
*Carbohydrate:* **39g** | *Dietary Fiber:* **7g**
*Protein:* **11g**

HEALTH BENEFITS:

# Cumin Quinoa

*Total time:* **25 minutes** | *Serves* **3**

INGREDIENTS:

2½ cups water
1 cup uncooked quinoa
1 tablespoon cumin
½ teaspoon turmeric powder
1 teaspoon salt
1 teaspoon extra-virgin coconut oil
   (or extra-virgin olive oil)
1 teaspoon black pepper
Dash cayenne pepper, if you like
   a little kick

ACTIONS:

1. In a pot, add the quinoa to 2½ cups of
   water. Bring to a boil over high heat.
2. Reduce heat to low, cover, and simmer
   for 15 minutes. The quinoa will absorb
   the water during the process.
3. Add the remaining ingredients and
   continue to cook, stirring occasionally,
   for another 3 minutes, or until the
   quinoa is soft and all flavors are well
   combined.

TIP:

Try using sesame seed oil instead of
coconut oil for a different flavor.

VARIATIONS:

1. Serve with avocado, cubed cucumber,
   a sprig of fresh parsley and cilantro,
   and a squeeze of lemon for Greens and
   Cumin Quinoa.
2. Serve with strawberries for Strawberry
   Cumin Quinoa!

*Calories:* **226** | *Total Fat:* **5g**
*Carbohydrate:* **39g** | *Dietary Fiber:* **4g**
*Protein:* **11g**

HEALTH BENEFITS:

# Coconut Basil Sweet Potato Fries

*Total time:* **20 minutes**  |  *Serves* **4**

## INGREDIENTS:

⅓ cup extra-virgin coconut oil

2 large sweet potatoes, cut into the shape of French fries

½ cup fresh basil (or dried basil)

½ cup dried, shredded coconut

## ACTIONS:

1. Heat the coconut oil in a frying pan.
2. When pan is sizzling add the sweet potato fries, stirring until each is coated with oil.
3. Let cook, flipping periodically, until they are golden brown (after 3–5 minutes).
4. After the fries have browned, gradually add basil and shredded coconut. Continue cooking until desired crunchiness (or softness) is achieved.

## TIPS:

1. To get closer to nature, shred your own coconut from the meat of a fresh coconut.
2. Sprinkle 1 teaspoon salt over cooked fries.
3. Sprinkle 1 tablespoon curry powder over cooked fries.

*Calories:* **484**  |  *Total Fat:* **45g**
*Carbohydrate:* **22g**  |  *Dietary Fiber:* **5g**
*Protein:* **3g**

## HEALTH BENEFITS:

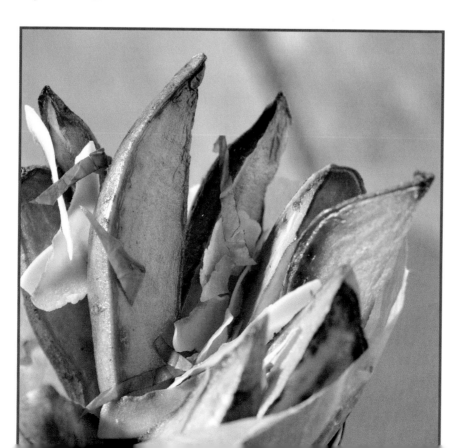

# Lentil Soup

*Total time:* **45 minutes** | *Serves* **4**

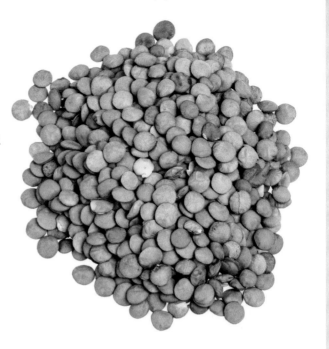

## INGREDIENTS:

5 tablespoons extra-virgin coconut oil
1 yellow onion, chopped
3 cloves garlic, chopped
½-inch piece ginger, chopped
2 teaspoons cumin
1 teaspoon dried thyme
1 teaspoon sage
1 teaspoon oregano
1 teaspoon turmeric powder
⅛ teaspoon cayenne pepper or more
   to taste
1 teaspoon salt
¼ teaspoon black pepper
6 cups water
1½ cup lentils
3 stalks celery, cut in ¼-inch slices
1 carrot, cut in ¼-inch slices
Juice of one lemon
4 tablespoons fresh chopped cilantro

## ACTIONS:

1. Heat the coconut oil in a large pot and add the onion and garlic. Sauté until golden brown (about 4 minutes). Add the ginger and stir-fry for one minute. Add the cumin, thyme, sage, oregano, and turmeric powder. Stir-fry for one minute more. Add cayenne pepper, salt, and black pepper. Stir-fry for another minute until the spices are fragrant.
2. Stir in the water, lentils, celery, and carrot. Bring to a boil over high heat then reduce to medium-low, cover, and simmer for 30 minutes or until lentils are soft.
3. Stir in the lemon and cilantro, and serve. Drizzle with olive oil and sprinkle with more salt or cayenne pepper to taste!

## TIPS:

1. Serve with Quick Bread (see p. 132).
2. Serve with rice or quinoa.
3. If you want a smoother, less chunky soup, puree the soup in a blender once cooked.
4. Some lentils are smaller than others and will require less cooking time.
5. For the busy lifestyle this is a good recipe to freeze and take out the day you need it.

## VARIATIONS:

1. Add 2 chopped tomatoes and 1 tablespoon tomato paste when adding the water for Tomato Lentil Soup.
2. Add 1½ tablespoons curry powder for Curry Lentil Soup.

*Calories:* **279** | *Total Fat:* **19g**
*Carbohydrate:* **24g** | *Dietary Fiber:* **13g**
*Protein:* **20g**

## HEALTH BENEFITS:

# Mushroom Soup

*Total time:* **35 minutes** | *Serves* **4**

### INGREDIENTS:

4 tablespoons Vegan Butter (see p. 147)

2 yellow onions, chopped

1 pound any kind of fresh mushrooms, sliced

2 teaspoons dill

1 tablespoon paprika

2 cups water

1 teaspoon salt

1 teaspoon thyme

1 cup nut or Seed Milk (see p. 86)

3 tablespoons diatomaceous earth, rice flour, or buckwheat flour

Ground black pepper to taste

2 teaspoons lemon juice (from ½ a lemon)

¼ cup fresh parsley, chopped

½ cup Vegan Sour Cream (see p. 151)

### ACTIONS:

1. In a large pot over medium heat, melt the butter. Sauté the onions in the butter for 3 minutes. Add the mushrooms and sauté for another 5 minutes.

2. Stir in the dill, paprika, water, salt, and thyme and continue cooking.

3. In a separate bowl, whisk the milk and diatomaceous earth together. Pour this into the soup, stir well to blend ingredients, and cover and simmer for 15 minutes. Stir occasionally.

4. Reduce the heat to low and stir in the black pepper, lemon juice, parsley, and sour cream. Mix together and allow to cook for another 5 minutes. Serve.

### TIPS:

1. Serve with Quick Bread (see p. 132).

2. Serve with rice or quinoa.

3. If you want a smoother, less chunky soup, puree the soup in a blender once cooked.

*Calories:* **333** | *Total Fat:* **27g**
*Carbohydrate:* **19g** | *Dietary Fiber:* **5g**
*Protein:* **10g**

### HEALTH BENEFITS:

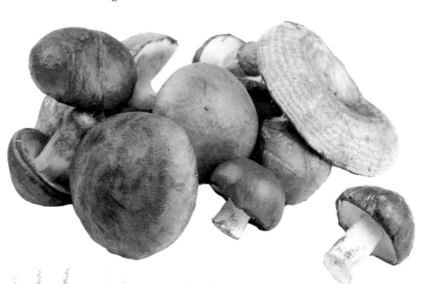

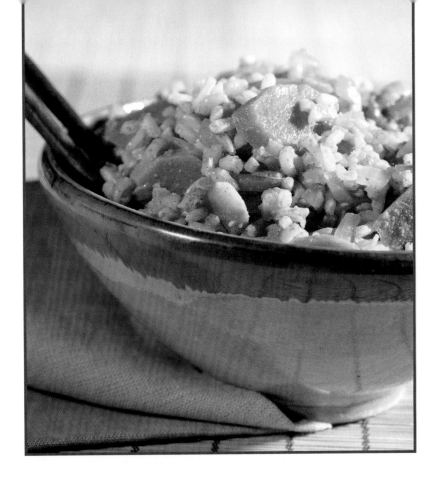

# Turmeric Rice

*Total time:* **45 minutes** | *Serves* **4**

### INGREDIENTS:

2 cups uncooked brown rice
2 tablespoons extra-virgin coconut oil
1 yellow onion, chopped
2 tablespoons chopped garlic
2 tablespoons turmeric powder
1 tablespoon chopped ginger
1 carrot, cut in finely sliced rounds

### ACTIONS:

1. Boil the rice in four cups of water, until slightly tender but not entirely cooked, approximately 30 minutes.
2. Heat the coconut oil in a frying pan on medium heat and fry the onion, garlic, turmeric powder, ginger, and carrots until they are golden brown and well combined.
3. Add the semi-cooked rice to the frying pan and stir-fry with the carrot mixture for 2 minutes, until the rice is done and has turned yellow from the turmeric.

### VARIATION:

Wrap a scoop of turmeric rice in a piece of lettuce for a Rice Taco.

*Calories:* **437** | *Total Fat:* **10g**
*Carbohydrate:* **79g** | *Dietary Fiber:* **5g**
*Protein:* **8g**

### HEALTH BENEFITS:

# Vegetable Stir-Fry

*Total time:* **35 minutes** | *Serves* **4**

## INGREDIENTS:

¼ cup extra-virgin coconut oil
1 yellow onion, chopped
4 large garlic cloves, chopped
1-inch piece ginger, chopped
1 teaspoon turmeric powder
½ teaspoon cumin
½ teaspoon thyme
¼ teaspoon salt
1 large carrot, chopped
½ a head of broccoli, chopped
½ a head of cauliflower, chopped
1 cup of spinach
1 cup green beans
1 tablespoon sesame seeds

## ACTIONS:

1. Heat the oil in a wok or frying pan and add onion and garlic. Sauté for two minutes then add ginger. Sauté for another minute then add turmeric powder, cumin, thyme, and salt.
2. Add the vegetables to the pan and stir-fry until tender about 10–15 minutes.
3. Serve, sprinkling sesame seeds over each dish, along with salt and pepper to taste.

## TIPS:

1. Serve with rice or quinoa.
2. Add other vegetables like peppers, snow peas, zucchini, beets, or peas.
3. Add your favorite spices for different flavors and added health benefits.
4. Add a squeeze of lemon right before serving for added health benefits.

## VARIATIONS:

1. Add 1½ cups of cooked brown rice pasta for Vegetable Pasta Stir-Fry.
2. Add 1 cup of cooked rice for Vegetable Rice Stir Fry.
3. Use sesame seed oil instead of coconut oil for Sesame Vegetable Stir-Fry.
4. Add ½ teaspoon or more cayenne pepper for Spicy Vegetable Stir-Fry.
5. Add 1 tablespoon or more of honey or maple syrup when adding the vegetables for Sweet Vegetable Stir-Fry.
6. If you are a meat eater you could add chicken, beef, or scrambled eggs to this dish for Meat and Veg Stir-Fry.
7. Add artichokes for Artichoke Vegetable Stir-Fry.

*Calories:* **190** | *Total Fat:* **16g**
*Carbohydrate:* **11g** | *Dietary Fiber:* **5g**
*Protein:* **5g**

## HEALTH BENEFITS:

DETOX  ANTI-INFLAM.  DH  ENERGY  IMMUNE BOOST

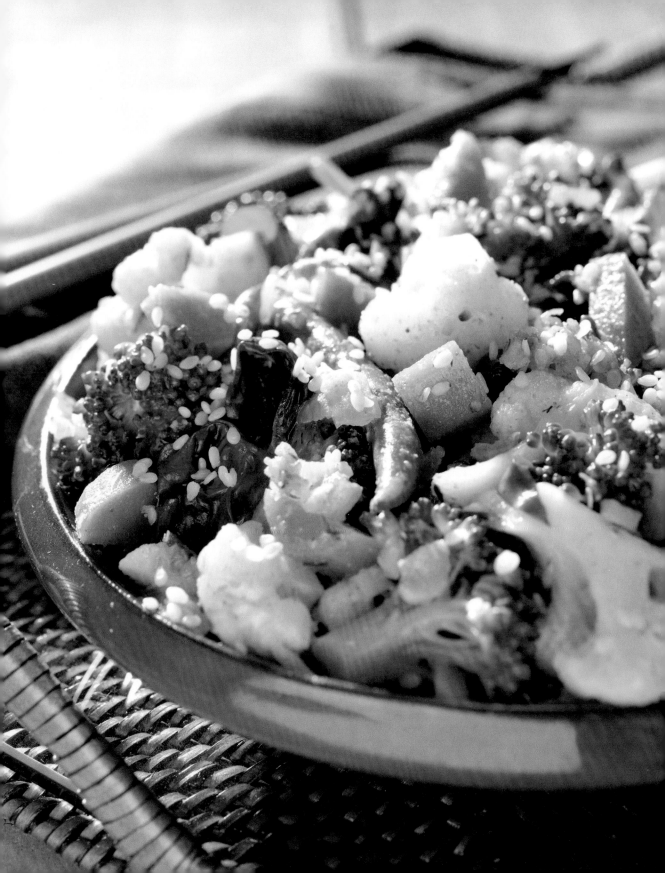

# Vegan Curry

*Total time:* **1 hour and 10 minutes** | *Serves* **4**

Served over rice or quinoa, or eat alone.

## INGREDIENTS:

2 tablespoons extra-virgin olive oil

1 yellow onion, diced

4 garlic cloves, chopped

5 large potatoes, chopped into 1-inch cubes

1 sweet potato, chopped into 1-inch cubes

1½ tablespoons curry powder

1 teaspoon fresh sage

1 teaspoon salt

½ teaspoon cayenne pepper

1 teaspoon chili powder, or diced fresh
    chili pepper

Juice of 1 lime

1½ cups coconut milk

1 teaspoon maple syrup

4 cups water

1 cup green beans, chopped in thirds
    and stems removed

## ACTIONS:

1. Heat the olive oil in a deep pot, and add the
   onion and garlic. Sauté until golden brown,
   about 3 minutes.
2. Add remaining ingredients, except green
   beans, to the pot. Simmer for 45 minutes,
   or until the potatoes are soft.
3. Add the green beans and cook another
   5 minutes, so beans remain crunchy.
4. Season with additional salt and black
   pepper to taste.

## TIP:

Make your own Coconut Milk (see p. 86)
instead of using a canned variety.

## VARIATION:

Add more cayenne pepper for
Spicy Vegan Curry.

*Calories:* **692** | *Total Fat:* **29g**
*Carbohydrate:* **106g** | *Dietary Fiber:* **16g**
*Protein:* **13g**

## HEALTH BENEFITS:

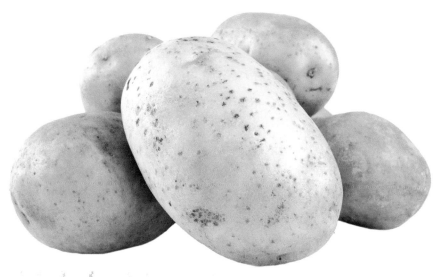

# Mashed Potatoes

*Total time:* **20 minutes** | *Serves* **2**

### INGREDIENTS:

2 large potatoes

3 tablespoons extra-virgin coconut oil
(or extra-virgin olive oil)

Ground black pepper and salt, to taste

### ACTIONS:

1. Boil the potatoes until they are completely soft.
2. Drain the water, and add the oil to the pot and mash potatoes.
3. Season to taste with salt and pepper.

### TIPS:

1. For even creamier mashed potatoes, replace the oil with Almond Milk (p. 85) or Seed Milk (p. 86).
2. If you want the mash to be smoother, add more oil or milk.

### VARIATIONS:

1. Replace the white potatoes with sweet potatoes for Mashed Sweet Potatoes.
2. Add ⅛ teaspoon or more cayenne pepper for Spicy Mashed Potatoes.

*Calories:* **401** | *Total Fat:* **14g**
*Carbohydrate:* **68g** | *Dietary Fiber:* **8g**
*Protein:* **7g**

### HEALTH BENEFITS:

# Vegan Soup

*Total time:* **2 hours** | *Serves* **4**

### INGREDIENTS:

1 yellow onion

2 large potatoes

2 large carrots

2 stalks celery

1 pound pumpkin or sweet potato

½ head broccoli

2 zucchinis

1 tablespoon extra-virgin olive oil

6 cloves garlic, crushed

5 cups water

½ tablespoon salt

1 tablespoon fresh sage or 1 teaspoon dried sage

### ACTIONS:

1. Dice the onion, potatoes, carrots, celery, pumpkin, broccoli, and zucchini into ½-inch cubes and set aside.
2. Over medium heat, add the olive oil to a large saucepan. Sauté the onion, celery, and garlic in the oil until the onions become transparent.
3. Add the remainder of the diced vegetables and the water, salt, and sage to the saucepan and bring to a boil. Simmer over medium heat for 90 minutes until the vegetables are broken down.
4. Season with additional salt and pepper to taste.

### VARIATION:

For more protein, add 2 cups dried beans of any kind (soaked for at least 12 hours) for Vegan Bean Soup.

*Calories:* **279** | *Total Fat:* **4g**
*Carbohydrate:* **58g** | *Dietary Fiber:* **10g**
*Protein:* **9g**

### HEALTH BENEFITS:

# Quick Bread

*Total time:* **15 minutes** | *Makes* **6**

## INGREDIENTS:

1½ cups rice flour
1½ cups buckwheat flour
1 cup warm water
2 teaspoons apple cider vinegar
1 tablespoon Flax Egg Alternative
   (see p. 150)

## ACTIONS:

1. Put the flours in a large bowl and while stirring, slowly add the water and vinegar. When that is combined, add the Flax Egg Alternative, forming the dough.
2. Once well mixed, knead the dough for two minutes until the dough feels tougher, and form into a ball.
3. Roll out the ball of dough with a rolling pin to make six 6-inch circles (⅓ cup of dough each).
4. Heat a cast-iron pan on medium heat on the stove, and once hot, place the flat bread in it. Cover the pan while it cooks (important for the softness of the bread). Cook for a minute or two on each side until there is no more soft dough.
5. Once the bread is ready, transfer to a plate and cover with a clean dish towel or cotton napkin to keep it soft. It is best eaten the day of preparation.

## TIPS:

1. Add 1 teaspoon of salt for enhanced flavor.
2. These can be used as wraps, sliced into pieces and dipped into hummus, or used as a pizza base!
3. This can also be made with whole wheat flour for people who can have gluten.

## VARIATION:

Add 1 teaspoon cayenne pepper for Spicy Quick Bread.

*Calories:* **250** | *Total Fat:* **3g**
*Carbohydrate:* **52g** | *Dietary Fiber:* **5g**
*Protein:* **7g**

## HEALTH BENEFITS:

# Gluten-free Rolls

*Total time:* **90 minutes to prepare dough, 15 minutes to bake** | *Makes* **6 bread rolls**

These rolls are best eaten the day they are made. They aren't as fresh the next day.

### INGREDIENTS:

2 packages of baker's yeast (10g total)
2 tablespoons maple syrup
½ cup lukewarm water
1 cup rice flour
1 cup buckwheat flour
1 teaspoon salt
1 tablespoon extra-virgin olive oil

### ACTIONS:

1. Put the yeast, maple syrup, and water into a cup. Stir, cover, and allow to sit in a warm place for 10 minutes.
2. Sift the rice flour and buckwheat flour into a glass bowl that is at warm room temperature, and then sprinkle with salt. Mix until well combined.
3. Make a well in the middle of the flour, then pour the yeast mixture into the well and begin combining. Form into soft dough.
4. Turn your dough onto a floured board and knead well, for at least 5 minutes. Kneading allows air in the bread. Form into one ball.
5. Oil a large bowl with extra-virgin olive oil. Place the dough (un-creased, or smooth side up) into the bowl and rub oil over the dough.
6. Cover the bowl with a cotton cloth and put in a warm place. Leave until the dough has doubled in size, 30 minutes to 1 hour.
7. Turn your dough onto a floured board and knead again for 5 minutes until a tough consistency is achieved. Divide the dough into six equal parts and knead each of these into a ball.

8. Place the dough balls close together on a lightly oiled baking sheet. Place uncovered in a warm spot and allow to rise again by ¼ inch, approximately 10–20 minutes. Preheat oven to 465°F while you wait for the dough to rise again.
9. Bake for 5 minutes. Reduce heat to 180°F and bake for another 5–10 minutes, until the rolls have risen and are slightly golden brown.

### TIP:

Make sure the yeast does not contain wheat gluten.

### VARIATIONS:

1. To make one entire loaf of bread, instead of dividing the bread into parts in Step 7, make one large ball of dough and then flatten it with your hand until it looks more like a flattened dome. Bake as the recipe instructs.
2. For those of you who are not concerned about consuming gluten, and if you want a softer bread roll, replace the buckwheat and rice flour with whole-wheat flour and proceed to follow the rest of the recipe as is for Whole Wheat Rolls.

*Calories:* **224** | *Total Fat:* **4g**
*Carbohydrate:* **44g** | *Dietary Fiber:* **4g**
*Protein:* **5g**

### HEALTH BENEFITS:

# CHAPTER 13

# Meat Eaters' Main Dishes

Baked Crusted Salmon

> ## "The best thing you can have in the kitchen is confidence."
> —Gordon Ramsay

# Baked Lamb Chops

*Total time:* **50 minutes**  |  *Serves* **3**

### INGREDIENTS:

12 5.5 ounce lamb chops or 6 large chops
2 ½ tablespoons extra-virgin olive oil
1 tablespoon garlic powder
1 tablespoon turmeric powder
1 tablespoon cumin powder
1½ teaspoons salt
1½ teaspoons pepper
1 cup walnuts blended into a meal

### ACTIONS:

1. Preheat oven to 375°F.
2. In a medium bowl, combine the garlic powder, turmeric, cumin, salt, pepper, and walnut meal.
3. Brush oil on both sides of each lamb chop. Dip the chops into the walnut mixture and then arrange them on a 9 x 13 inch baking dish. Sprinkle additional walnut mixture on the chops, covering them as much as possible.
4. Bake in the oven for 20 minutes. Turn the chops over and cook for another 20 minutes.

### TIPS:

1. Serve with Mashed Potatoes or Coconut Basil Sweet Potato Fries.
2. Use eggs to make the coating stick to the lamb chops better. Whisk 2 eggs, then dip the chops in, and then coat them with the walnut mixture.

### VARIATION:

You can cook the lamb chops in a frying pan instead of the oven to save time. They will be ready in less than 8 minutes, about 4 minutes on each side. Follow the same directions as above, except heat a frying pan with oil and then cook for Fried Lamb Chops.

*Calories:* **538**  |  *Total Fat:* **50g**
*Carbohydrate:* **8g**  |  *Dietary Fiber:* **5g**
*Protein:* **16g**

### HEALTH BENEFITS:

# Beef Stir-Fry

*Total time:* **1–4 hours marinating, 20 minutes cooking** | *Serves* **4**

Serve the stir-fry over a bed of rice or quinoa.

## INGREDIENTS:

1 cup freshly squeezed orange juice

2 tablespoons water

2 teaspoons chopped ginger

1 garlic clove, chopped

½ teaspoon cayenne pepper

1 pound boneless sirloin steak, cut into thin strips

1 tablespoon extra-virgin coconut oil

5 cups chopped vegetables, such as broccoli, sugar snap peas, red bell peppers, cabbage, carrots

1 tablespoon raw honey

1 teaspoon sesame seeds

## ACTIONS:

1. Make the marinade by mixing the orange juice, water, ginger, garlic, and cayenne pepper in a large bowl.

2. Place the beef in the bowl with the marinade, making sure each strip of beef is well coated. Cover the bowl and marinate for 1–4 hours in the refrigerator.

3. Heat the coconut oil in a large skillet over medium heat.

4. Add the marinated beef to the skillet and stir-fry for 4 minutes, until beef is no longer pink.

5. Remove the beef strips from the skillet and drizzle the honey over strips. Allow to sit until you return the beef to the skillet in Step 7.

6. Add the chopped vegetables to the same skillet and stir-fry them for 3–5 minutes.

7. Return the beef to the skillet and stir-fry everything together for 2 minutes to marry the flavors.

8. Sprinkle sesame seeds over stir-fry before serving.

*Calories:* **368** | *Total Fat:* **21g**
*Carbohydrate:* **21g** | *Dietary Fiber:* **3g**
*Protein:* **26g**

## HEALTH BENEFITS:

PROTEIN AO DH ANTI-INFLAM. IMMUNE BOOST

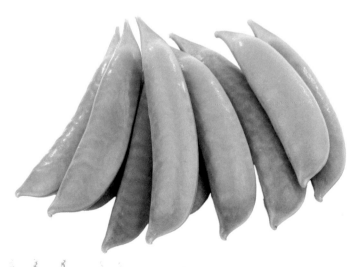

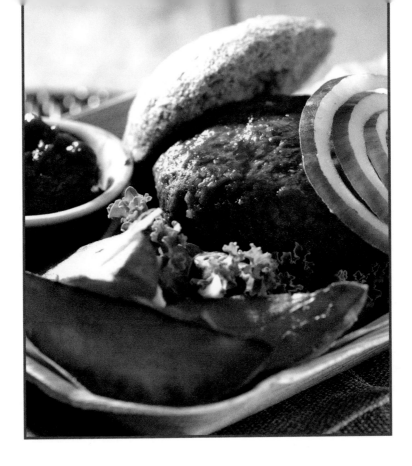

# Burgers

*Total time:* **20 minutes** | *Serves* **4**

## INGREDIENTS:

1 pound ground beef

2 eggs, beaten

1 cup almond meal

1 tablespoon fresh sage, or 1 teaspoon
   dried sage

2 teaspoons salt

1 teaspoon cumin

1 teaspoon turmeric powder

½ teaspoon black pepper

¼ cup extra-virgin coconut oil

## ACTIONS:

1. In a large bowl, combine all the
   ingredients, except the coconut oil.
   Mix until thoroughly combined.

2. Form four patties by hand.

3. Heat a large frying pan with the coconut oil
   over medium heat. When the pan is hot,
   place the patties in it.

4. Allow the patties to cook until the
   underside has browned, then flip over.
   Cook until desired doneness is achieved.

## TIPS:

1. Serve with lettuce as the wrap, or on
   Gluten-free Rolls (see p. 133).

2. Accompany with French Fries (see p. 119).

3. Top with Ketchup (see p. 150).

*Calories:* **503** | *Total Fat:* **42g**
*Carbohydrate:* **6g** | *Dietary Fiber:* **3g**
*Protein:* **30g**

## HEALTH BENEFITS:

# Chicken Nuggets

*Total time:* **30 minutes** | *Serves* **4**

## INGREDIENTS:

1 pound boneless, skinless chicken breasts
1 cup whole almonds
2 tablespoons turmeric powder
2 teaspoons salt
2 eggs
¾ cup extra-virgin coconut oil

## ACTIONS:

1. In a blender, mix the almonds, turmeric powder, and salt until the mixture has a fine flour meal consistency. Some chunks are okay. Place on a plate.
2. Cut the chicken breast into nugget-sized pieces.
3. Crack the eggs into a bowl and whisk with a fork.
4. Dip the chicken in the egg, coating well.
5. Dredge chicken in flour meal, coating well on all sides.
6. Heat the coconut oil in a frying pan over medium heat. When the oil is hot, carefully place the chicken pieces in the pan one by one. Let one side of the chicken cook until golden brown and crispy. Flip the nuggets and cook the other side.
7. Carefully remove the chicken from the oil. Place on a towel to absorb excess oil if you like, then serve.

## TIP:

Serve with Coconut Basil Sweet Potato Fries (see p. 124) and Green Salad (see p. 106).

## VARIATIONS:

1. For extra heat, add 1 teaspoon or more cayenne pepper to the flour meal mixture for Spicy Chicken Nuggets.
2. Use fish for Fish Fingers.
3. Coat a whole chicken breast fillet in the flour meal for Chicken Schnitzel.
4. Coat a quarter pound of beef fillet for Beef Schnitzel.
5. Cut a chicken breast fillet in half and sprinkle nutritional yeast inside. Put the chicken back together, then coat in flour meal for Chicken Cordon Bleu.
6. Cut a chicken breast fillet in half and add 2 tablespoons Vegan Butter with 1 garlic clove, chopped, then put the chicken back together and coat with flour meal for Chicken Kiev.

*Calories:* **724** | *Total Fat:* **62g**
*Carbohydrate:* **10g** | *Dietary Fiber:* **5g**
*Protein:* **36g**

## HEALTH BENEFITS:

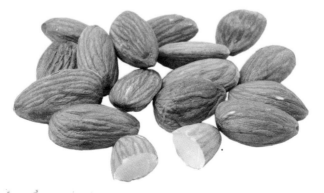

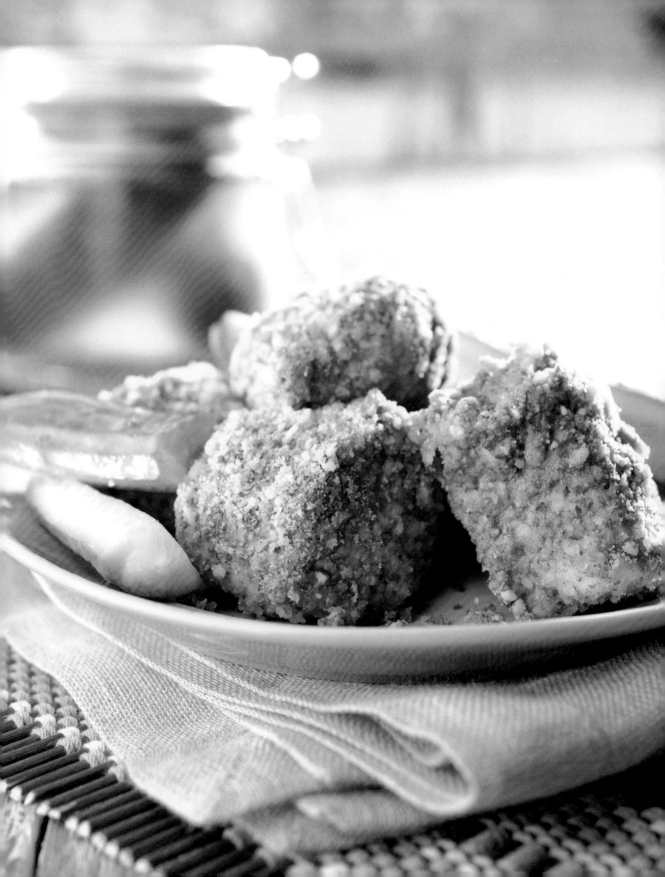

# Beef Burritos

*Total time:* **25 minutes** | *Serves* **6**
**(1 burrito each)**

## INGREDIENTS:

1 pound ground beef
1 tablespoon extra-virgin coconut oil
1 small yellow onion, chopped
2 large garlic cloves, diced
1½ teaspoons ground cumin
½ teaspoon turmeric powder
¼ teaspoon salt
¼ teaspoon pepper
1 teaspoon chili powder or ¼ teaspoon
    cayenne pepper (optional if you want it
    a little spicy)
6 brown rice tortillas/wraps or Quick Bread
    (see p. 132)
Toppings of your choice: 3¼ cup Vegan Sour
    Cream (see p. 151), 1 cup nutritional yeast,
    ½ cup grated carrot, diced lettuce,
    1 avocado cubed, 1 diced pepper,
    fresh cilantro, Ketchup (see p. 150),
    and/or 16 ounces black beans (soaked,
    cooked, soft).

## ACTIONS:

1. Heat a large frying pan with oil and cook
   the beef over medium heat for 3–4 minutes
   or until it turns brown, stirring frequently.
2. Add the onion, garlic, chili powder, cumin,
   turmeric powder, salt, and pepper to
   meat and stir. Cook for 7 minutes
   or until the vegetables are tender
   and flavors are well combined.
3. Place ¼ cup of meat into each
   tortilla and then fill the rest
   with your toppings!

## TIPS:

1. If you want to take it a step further,
   heat the oven to 375°F, place burritos on
   parchment paper, and bake for 12 minutes,
   until the burritos have turned golden
   brown.
2. Add ¼ cup Ketchup (see p. 150) to
   the beef.

## VARIATIONS:

1. Use chicken for Chicken Burritos.
2. Use fish for Fish Burritos.
3. Use beans and Vegetable Stir-Fry
   for Veggie Burritos.

*Calories:* **204** | *Total Fat:* **8g**
*Carbohydrate:* **10g** | *Dietary Fiber:* **1g**
*Protein:* **22g**

## HEALTH BENEFITS:

PROTEIN ENERGY ANTI-INFLAM. AO DH

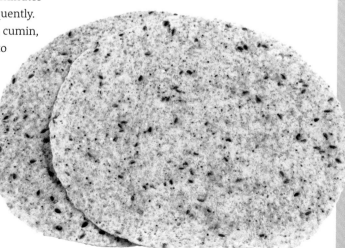

# Caramel Shrimp

*Total time:* **10 minutes** | *Serves* **4**

## INGREDIENTS:

¼ cup extra-virgin coconut oil
1 pound raw shrimp, peeled and
   deveined
3 tablespoons raw honey

## ACTIONS:

1. Heat the coconut oil in a frying pan over medium heat. When hot, add the shrimp.
2. After a minute, drizzle half of the honey over the shrimp.
3. Continue to cook for 3–5 minutes— stirring occasionally—until the shrimp turns opaque and is cooked through. Drizzle the rest of the honey over the shrimp 20 seconds before removing from the pan.

## TIPS:

1. Serve with a Green Salad (see p. 106) and French Fries (see p. 119).
2. Replace the honey with maple syrup for another sweet alternative.

## VARIATION:

Add ½ teaspoon of cayenne pepper, for Spicy Caramel Shrimp.

*Calories:* **284** | *Total Fat:* **16g**
*Carbohydrate:* **14g** | *Dietary Fiber:* **0g**
*Protein:* **23g**

## HEALTH BENEFITS:

# Omelet

*Total time:* **10 minutes** | *Serves* **2**

## INGREDIENTS:

5 eggs
3 tablespoons extra-virgin coconut oil
Black pepper and salt, to taste

## ACTIONS:

1. Crack the eggs into a bowl and whisk with a fork.
2. Heat the coconut oil in a frying pan over medium heat. Make sure that the oil covers the entire bottom of the pan; if not, add more oil. When the oil is hot, pour in the eggs.
3. Cook until top begins to firm, then flip.
4. Cook on the other side until desired doneness is achieved.

## TIP:

Serve with avocado slices.

## VARIATIONS:

1. Add ½ teaspoon cayenne pepper for Spicy Eggs.
2. Add 2 tablespoons nutritional yeast for Cheesy Eggs.
3. Add 2 tablespoons chopped green onions and 2 tablespoons fresh cilantro for Eggs with Greens.
4. Serve on Quick Bread for Egg Wraps.

*Calories:* **393** | *Total Fat:* **38g**
*Carbohydrate:* **1g** | *Dietary Fiber:* **0g**
*Protein:* **14g**

## HEALTH BENEFITS:

# Fish and Chips

*Total time:* **30 minutes** | *Serves* **4**

## INGREDIENTS:

4 small potatoes

¾ cup extra-virgin coconut oil

1 egg

1 cup almond meal

¾ teaspoon salt

1 teaspoon turmeric powder

4 small pieces fish (try salmon, whiting,
   or bass)

## ACTIONS:

1. Cut the potatoes into the shape of
   French fries.
2. Heat ½ cup of the coconut oil over medium
   heat in a large frying pan. When the oil is
   hot and starting to sizzle, add the potatoes.
3. Cook the potatoes until they are golden
   brown on one side and flip. Remove when
   done and drain on paper towels.
4. While the fries are cooking, make the fish
   coating. Crack the egg into a shallow bowl
   and whisk with a fork.
5. In another shallow bowl, combine the
   almond meal, salt, and turmeric powder.
6. Dredge the fish in the egg and coat well.
   Dredge fish in almond-meal mixture and
   coat well on both sides.
7. Heat remaining ¼ cup coconut oil in
   another frying pan. When the oil is hot,
   place the fish in it. Cook for 3–5 minutes
   on each side, flipping when golden brown.
   Remove when done and serve with the
   fries. Place on a towel to remove excess oil
   if you feel it necessary.

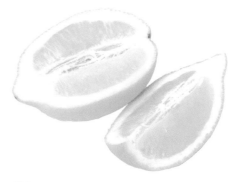

## TIP:

Serve with lemon wedges.

## VARIATION:

Add ½ teaspoon cayenne pepper to the
almond mix for Spicy Fish and Chips.

*Calories:* **758** | *Total Fat:* **59g**
*Carbohydrate:* **37g** | *Dietary Fiber:* **7g**
*Protein:* **27g**

## HEALTH BENEFITS:

# Baked Crusted Salmon

*Total time:* **35 minutes** | *Serves* **4**

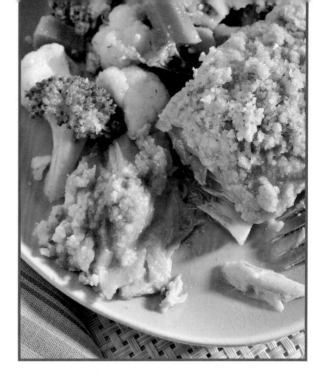

### INGREDIENTS:

1½ pounds of skinless salmon,
    cut into 4 pieces
1 cup walnuts blended to a meal
1 teaspoon sage
1 teaspoon thyme
½ teaspoon salt
4 tablespoons coconut oil

### ACTIONS:

1. Preheat oven to 380°F.
   Prepare a baking sheet with
   parchment paper or thin coating
   of coconut oil.
2. Mix the walnut meal, sage, thyme,
   and salt in a bowl. Brush the fillets with oil.
   Press each fillet into the walnut mixture to
   coat on both sides. Place the salmon on the
   baking sheet.
3. Bake for 7 minutes, turn the salmon over,
   and bake for another 7 minutes, or to your
   desired doneness.

### TIPS:

1. Serve this with roasted potatoes, French
   Fries (see p. 119), Green Salad (see p. 106),
   and/or Mashed Potatoes (see p. 131).
2. Use one beaten egg to help the coating stick
   to the salmon. Dip the salmon in the egg
   and then coat with walnut mixture.
3. For fewer calories, place the salmon
   on the baking sheet and sprinkle your
   desired amount of walnut mixture on
   top and bake.
4. Use almonds, pecans, brazil nuts, or
   macadamia nuts instead of walnuts.
5. For a nut-free version, use ground-up
   hemp seeds, sunflower seeds, or pumpkin
   seeds instead of walnuts.

### VARIATIONS:

1. Drizzle with honey once cooked for
   Honey Baked Crusted Salmon.
2. Drizzle with honey and sprinkle with
   mustard seeds before serving the salmon
   for Honey Mustard Baked Crusted Salmon.
3. For a fried version, instead of baking,
   heat a frying pan with oil and cook for
   Fried Crusted Salmon.

*Calories:* **408** | *Total Fat:* **29g**
*Carbohydrate:* **12g** | *Dietary Fiber:* **5g**
*Protein:* **18g**

### HEALTH BENEFITS:

# Roast Chicken

*Total time:* **1 hour and 25 minutes** | *Serves* **4**

### INGREDIENTS:

1 whole chicken (about 3 pounds)
⅓ cup extra-virgin olive oil
1 teaspoon onion powder
1 teaspoon garlic powder
1 teaspoon thyme
1 teaspoon sage
½ teaspoon salt
½ teaspoon pepper

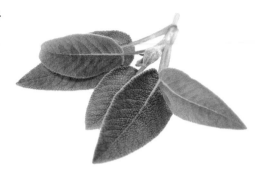

### ACTIONS:

1. Preheat the oven to 350°F.
2. Place the chicken in a roasting pan.
3. In a bowl mix the onion powder, garlic powder, thyme, sage, salt, and pepper to make the seasoning.
4. Coat the chicken in the olive oil, and sprinkle the seasoning mixture over the chicken.
5. Bake uncovered for 30 minutes, then take the chicken out of the oven and baste the chicken with the pan drippings.
6. Bake for another 30 minutes, then take the chicken out of the oven and baste the chicken with the pan drippings again.
7. Bake another 15 minutes or until the chicken is completely cooked through.

### TIPS:

1. Serve with Green Salad (see p. 106), French Fries (see p. 119), or Mashed Potatoes (see p. 131).
2. You can use any herbs you want in this recipe. For example oregano, basil, paprika, and rosemary work well.
3. Make stuffing by filling the center of the chicken with mixture of one cup of semi-cooked brown rice pasta or quinoa, 1 chopped celery stalk, 1 tablespoon oil, and 1 teaspoon thyme. Cook the chicken as instructed above.

### VARIATIONS:

1. Add 2 teaspoons turmeric powder to the seasoning for Roasted Turmeric Chicken.
2. For Roasted Garlic Chicken, chop 2 garlic cloves into four pieces each. Then cut small slits in the skin and insert the garlic pieces. Then season as above!
3. For Chicken with Roast Potatoes, cut potatoes into quarters, place them around the chicken, and bake with the chicken.
4. For Chicken with Gravy, when the chicken has finished cooking and has been removed from the pan to serve, add some buckwheat or rice flour and salt to the oil and stir for gravy. How much flour you need to add will depend on how much oil remains in the pan. Start with 1 teaspoon of flour and then keep adding until you reach the desired consistency.
5. For Smoky Roast Chicken, add 3 teaspoons paprika to the seasoning.

*Calories:* **259** | *Total Fat:* **9g**
*Carbohydrate:* **0g** | *Dietary Fiber:* **0g**
*Protein:* **42g**

### HEALTH BENEFITS:

# Honey-Rosemary Chicken

*Total time:* **15 minutes** | *Serves* **3,** makes 9 skewers

## INGREDIENTS:

1 pound boneless, skinless chicken breasts, cut into bite-size cubes
3 garlic cloves, diced
1 bunch fresh rosemary
5 tablespoons raw honey
¼ cup extra-virgin coconut oil, for frying

## ACTIONS:

1. Slide the rosemary leaves off from the stems. Reserve the stems for later. Dice the rosemary leaves.
2. In a large mixing bowl, stir together the garlic, rosemary leaves, and honey. Reserve 1 tablespoon for later use.
3. Place the chicken cubes in the bowl and stir until coated. Marinate 1–3 hours in the refrigerator or cook right away. Discard used marinade.
4. Put chicken pieces on reserved rosemary stems or wooden skewers.
5. Heat a frying pan with coconut oil— or fire up a grill! Once hot, cook the chicken until it is cooked through.
6. Drizzle the reserved marinade on the cooked chicken to serve.

## TIP:

Serve with French Fries (p. 119).

## VARIATION:

Wrap cooked chicken pieces in lettuce leaves for Honey-Rosemary Chicken Wraps.

*Calories:* **444** | *Total Fat:* **21g**
*Carbohydrate:* **32g** | *Dietary Fiber:* **1g**
*Protein:* **35g**

## HEALTH BENEFITS:

# Simple Sage Fish

*Total time:* **15 minutes** | *Serves* **1**

## INGREDIENTS:

1 tablespoon extra-virgin coconut oil
1 piece of fish, such as tuna steak, swordfish steak, salmon steak, or fillet just less than ½-inch thick
1 ½ teaspoons dried sage
1 lemon
Salt, to taste
Ground black pepper, to taste

## ACTIONS:

1. In a frying pan, heat the coconut oil on medium heat. Once hot, add the fish.
2. While the fish is cooking, sprinkle half of the sage and the juice of half the lemon over the fish.
3. Once you see half the fish is turning from raw to white from the bottom up, flip the fish. Sprinkle the remainder of the sage over the fish and cook through.
4. Remove the fish and plate. Squeeze remaining lemon juice onto fish. Season with salt and pepper to taste.

## TIP:

Serve with Green Salad (see p. 106), French Fries (see p. 119), or Mashed Potatoes (see p. 131).

## VARIATIONS:

1. Add 2 teaspoons garlic powder instead of sage for Simple Garlic Fish.
2. Add ½ teaspoon of thyme and oregano for Simple Herb Fish.
3. Add a dash of cayenne pepper on each side for Simple Spicy Fish.

*Calories:* **610** | *Total Fat:* **56g**
*Carbohydrate:* **6g** | *Dietary Fiber:* **1g**
*Protein:* **27g**

## HEALTH BENEFITS:

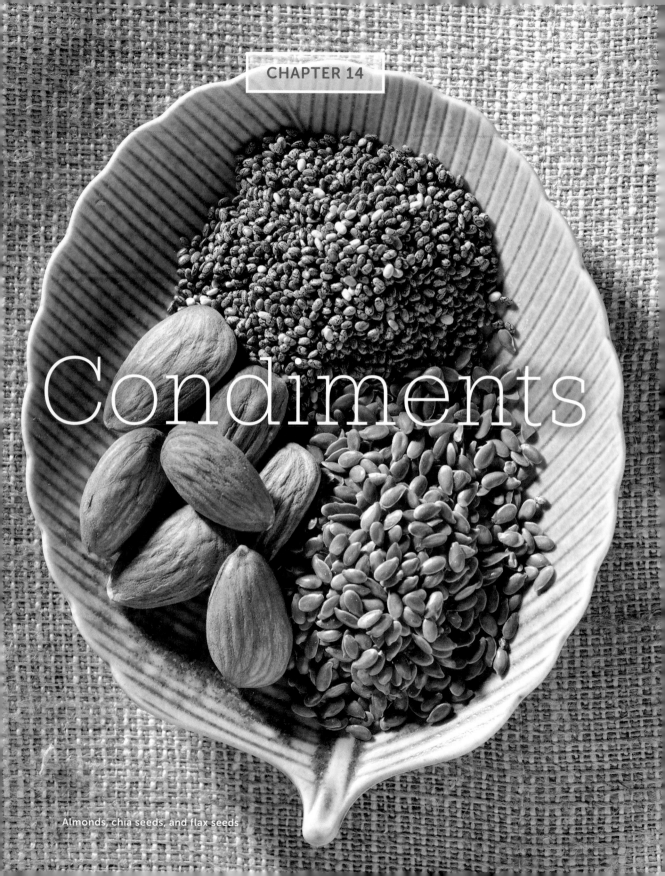

# CHAPTER 14

# Condiments

Almonds, chia seeds, and flax seeds

> **"Food is the basis of a joyful,
> happy life–a life worth relishing."**
>
> — Daphne Oz

# Vegan Butter

*Total time:* **25 minutes prep, 1 hour setting**
*Makes* **½ cup, 16 servings (½ tablespoon each)**

This butter can be stored in an airtight container in the refrigerator for up to one month. In a freezer, in a jar, this butter will last up to one year.

## INGREDIENTS:

¼ cup plus 2 teaspoons Almond Milk
   (see p. 85)
1 teaspoon apple cider vinegar
½ teaspoon salt
½ cup extra-virgin coconut oil, melted
1 tablespoon extra-virgin olive oil

## ACTIONS:

1. Place the Almond Milk, apple cider vinegar, and salt in a small cup and whisk together with a fork.
2. Let sit for ten minutes, until the mixture curdles.
3. Add the coconut oil and olive oil to a blender and mix on high speed until well combined and smooth.
4. Add the Almond Milk mixture. Mix for 2 minutes until smooth and creamy.
5. Place the mixture into a mold and place in the freezer to solidify. An ice cube tray works well as a mold. It will be ready to use as butter in one hour.

## TIPS:

1. To make your butter nut free, use Seed Milk (see p. 86) as an alternative to Almond Milk.
2. Other alternatives for toast or pancakes are extra-virgin coconut oil, extra-virgin olive oil, or avocado oil. You can also use avocado as a butter substitute.

## VARIATIONS:

1. Add ¼ teaspoon cinnamon and 2 teaspoons maple syrup to the oil for Cinnamon Butter.
2. Make Cinnamon Toast by spreading the Cinnamon Butter on Quick Bread or Gluten-free Rolls.

*Calories:* **70** | *Total Fat:* **8g**
*Carbohydrate:* **1g** | *Dietary Fiber:* **0g**
*Protein:* **1g**

## HEALTH BENEFITS:

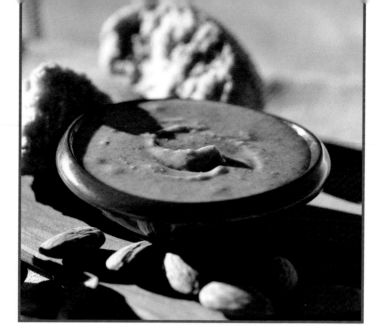

# Almond Butter

*Total time:* **30 minutes** | *Makes* **2 cups, serves 32 (1 tablespoon serving size)**

Almond Butter keeps in a jar with a shelf life of one month unrefrigerated. In the fridge, it is good for three months.

## INGREDIENT:

**3 cups raw or roasted almonds**

## ACTION:

Add the almonds to a food processor. (A food processor with an S-blade works best; a blener will not work well for this recipe.) Blend on high 20–30 minutes. The nuts will first become almond meal. Then, after about 15 or 20 minutes, the nut meal will release oils and eventually become a smooth almond butter—no other ingredient needed! It literally transforms from a dry meal into a smooth butter.

## VARIATIONS:

1. Substitute peanuts for the almonds for Peanut Butter.
2. Substitute walnuts for the almonds for Walnut Butter.
3. Substitute macadamias for almonds for Macadamia Butter.
4. Substitute cashews for almonds for Cashew Butter.
5. Substitute Brazil nuts for almonds for Brazil Nut Butter.
6. Substitute pecans for almonds for Pecan Butter.
7. Substitute hazelnuts for Hazelnut Butter.
8. Add 1 teaspoon of raw honey or maple syrup for Sweet Almond Butter.
9. Add 1 teaspoon of cacao powder for Chocolate Almond Butter.

*Calories:* **181** | *Total Fat:* **18g**
*Carbohydrate:* **4g** | *Dietary Fiber:* **2g**
*Protein:* **4g**

## HEALTH BENEFITS:

# Chia Seed Jam

*Total time:* **20 minutes** | *Serves* **12**

The jam will last up to two months in the refrigerator and six months in the freezer.

## INGREDIENTS:

**2 cups of your choice of berries, diced (strawberries work well)**
**1 cup water**
**¼ cup chia seeds**
**¼ cup maple syrup or honey**

## ACTIONS:

1. Place all ingredients into a pot and bring to a boil.
2. Reduce heat to a simmer and stir constantly so the chia seeds do not burn on the bottom of the pot.
3. When the mixture has thickened and the fruit is entirely broken down (about 10 minutes), allow to cool, and then place in a glass jar and cool completely before placing in the fridge. The jam is now ready to eat, but refrigerate overnight and the jam will set more. Serve on Gluten-free Rolls, or as a garnish for any of the desserts.

## VARIATIONS:

1. Use blueberries for Blueberry Chia Seed Jam.
2. Use blackberries for Blackberry Chia Seed Jam.
3. Use raspberries for Raspberry Chia Seed Jam.
4. Use mulberries for Mulberry Chia Seed Jam.
5. Use cranberries for Cranberry Chia Seed Jam.
6. Use ¼ cup each strawberries, blackberries, raspberries, and blueberries for Mixed Berry Chia Seed Jam.

*Calories:* **35** | *Total Fat:* **1g**
*Carbohydrate:* **7g** | *Dietary Fiber:* **1g**
*Protein:* **1g**

## HEALTH BENEFITS:

WEIGHT LOSS · DH · ANTI-INFLAM. · AO · IMMUNE BOOST

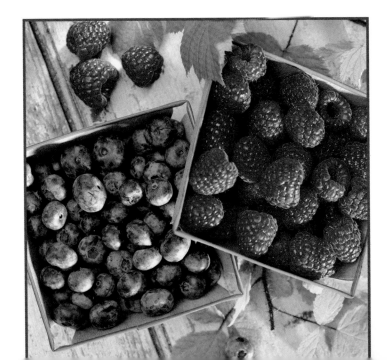

# Flax Egg Alternative

*Total time:* **10 minutes** | *For every egg in an original recipe, use one serving of this flax mix.*

*This is a great vegan alternative to egg.*

### INGREDIENTS:

3 teaspoons ground flaxseed
4 teaspoons water

### ACTIONS:

1. In a bowl, whisk the ingredients together.
2. Let sit for 5–10 minutes. It will become gummy, just like eggs.

*Calories:* **37** | *Total Fat:* **3g**
*Carbohydrate:* **2g** | *Dietary Fiber:* **2g**
*Protein:* **1g**

### HEALTH BENEFITS:

    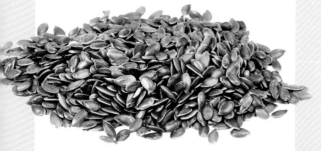

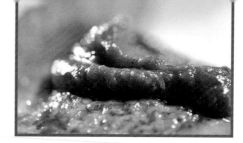

# Ketchup

*Total time:* **10 minutes** | *Makes* **3 cups**
**(48 1-tablespoon servings)**

Ketchup keeps well in the refrigerator for up to three months, or the freezer for six months.

### INGREDIENTS:

14 ounces organic tomato paste
1 ½ cups water
2 tablespoons maple syrup
3 teaspoons apple cider vinegar
⅓ tablespoon onion powder
⅔ teaspoon salt
½ teaspoon cinnamon
⅓ teaspoon garlic powder
Pinch of ground cloves
Dash of cayenne pepper

### ACTIONS:

1. Put all the ingredients into a blender and mix well.
2. Pour into a glass container and store in the fridge. Flavors will mesh well overnight.

### TIP:

Add a dash of nutmeg for added flavor.

### VARIATION:

Add 1 teaspoon dried mustard powder for Mustard Ketchup.

*Calories:* **7** | *Total Fat:* **0g**
*Carbohydrate:* **2g** | *Dietary Fiber:* **0g**
*Protein:* **0g**

### HEALTH BENEFITS:

# Salad Dressing

*Total time:* **5 minutes**  |  *Makes* **¼ cup dressing (for one large salad)**

Refrigerated in an airtight container or jar, this salad dressing lasts for up to two months.

## INGREDIENTS:

**2 cloves garlic, minced**
**1-inch piece ginger, minced**
**Juice of 1 lemon**
**¼ cup extra virgin olive oil**

## ACTIONS:

1. Add all the ingredients to a bowl and mix until well combined.
2. Pour on salad.

## VARIATIONS:

1. For Turmeric Salad Dressing, add 1 teaspoon turmeric powder, which gives extra health benefits.
2. Add 1 tablespoon honey or maple syrup for Sweet Salad Dressing.
3. Add ½ teaspoon cayenne pepper for Spicy Salad Dressing.
4. Add 1 avocado to the mixing bowl for a creamy dressing.
5. Add 1 tablespoon nutritional yeast to the dressing and mix for a Cheesy Dressing.
6. Add 2 tablespoons Hummus (see p. 120) for Hummus Salad Dressing.
7. Add 2 tablespoons Tahini (see p. 120) for Tahini Salad Dressing.
8. Add ¼ teaspoon mustard powder, 3 tablespoons nutritional yeast, and ½ teaspoon honey for Caesar Salad Dressing.

*Calories:* **100**  |  *Total Fat:* **11g**
*Carbohydrate:* **1g**  |  *Dietary Fiber:* **0g**
*Protein:* **0g**

## HEALTH BENEFITS:

# Vegan Sour Cream

*Total time:* **5 minutes**  |  *Makes* **1 cup, 8 servings**

Refrigerated in an airtight container or jar, this sour cream lasts for up to two weeks.

## INGREDIENTS:

**1 cup raw cashew nuts**
**¼ teaspoon salt**
**1 teaspoon apple cider vinegar**
**Juice of 1 small lemon (no more than ¼ cup)**
**½ teaspoon dill**
**3½ tablespoons water, or more if you need to make it smoother**

## ACTION:

Add all the ingredients to a blender and mix until the consistency is creamy.

## TIPS:

1. For a nut-free alternative, substitute sunflower seeds or hemp seeds for cashew nuts.
2. For a creamier sour cream, soak the cashews for four hours in water If you do soak the cashews, use half the amount of water in recipe.
3. Use this in any recipe that calls for sour cream.
4. Use this sour cream on Raw Tacos (see p. 113) and Raw Crackers (see p. 111).

*Calories:* **119**  |  *Total Fat:* **9g**
*Carbohydrate:* **7g**  |  *Dietary Fiber:* **1g**
*Protein:* **4g**

## HEALTH BENEFITS:

# CHAPTER 15

# Desserts

Raw Cashew Cheesecake

## "Life is uncertain. Eat dessert first."

— Ernestine Ulmer

# Raw Cashew Cheesecake

*Total time:* **3 hours to soak nuts, 25 minutes preparation, 4 hours freezing** | *Serves* **16**

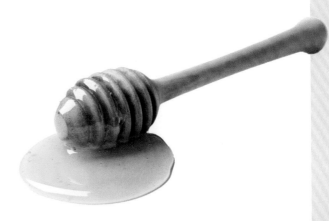

INGREDIENTS:

*For the Base*
4 cups almond meal
5 tablespoons maple syrup (or raw honey)
1 tablespoon coconut oil

*For the Cheesecake Filling*
½ cup lemon juice (approximately
   2 large lemons)
3 cups cashew nuts, soaked in water
   for 3 hours to soften
¾ cup maple syrup
¾ cup coconut oil
1 tablespoon pure vanilla extract
⅛ teaspoon salt

ACTIONS:

1. Make the base. In a bowl, combine the almond meal, maple syrup (or honey), and coconut oil. The mixture should be dry, but moist enough to hold together. Add a little water if the mixture is too dry.
2. Turn the base mixture into a deep pie dish (large enough to hold 2½ quarts) and press it evenly to cover the bottom and sides of dish. Set aside.
3. Make the cheesecake filling. Put all the ingredients in a powerful blender and blend until filling is very smooth and light in texture. Pour the filling into the prepared crust.
4. Freeze for 4 hours. Once set, cut into slices and serve.

TIP:
To make a smaller cheesecake, halve the recipe.

VARIATIONS:

1. Spoon 1 tablespoon of cheesecake filling into each of 32 paper baking cups for Mini Cheesecakes.
2. Top with a few fresh berries.

*Calories:* **368** | *Total Fat:* **28g**
*Carbohydrate:* **23g** | *Dietary Fiber:* **6g**
*Protein:* **10g**

HEALTH BENEFITS:

Desserts

# Apple Crumble

*Total time:* **30 minutes** | *Serves* **5**

## INGREDIENTS:

4 large apples, peeled, cored, and cut into
   bite-sized pieces
1 tablespoon extra-virgin coconut oil
1½ cups almond meal
⅓ cup dried, shredded coconut
2 tablespoons cinnamon powder
5 tablespoons maple syrup

## ACTIONS:

1. Preheat oven to 400°F.
2. Bring a pot of water to boil. Add the apple
   pieces and cook until they are semi soft.
3. In a small skillet over low heat, heat
   the coconut oil. Add the almond meal,
   shredded coconut, cinnamon, and
   2 tablespoons maple syrup and toast
   the mixture. Set aside for the time being.
4. Drain the water from the apple pieces and
   add the remaining 3 tablespoons maple
   syrup to the pot. Stir while continuing to
   cook the apples over medium-low heat,
   until the apples are soft. Remove from heat.
5. In an oven-proof dish, combine the apples
   with the toasted nut mixture. Bake for
   10 minutes.

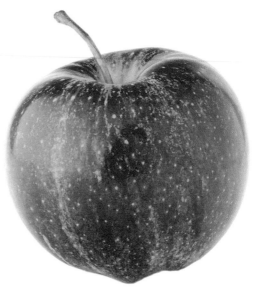

## TIPS:

1. This tastes delicious served with Vegan
   Ice Cream and chunks of nuts.
2. Substitute raw honey for the maple syrup
   if you prefer.

## VARIATION:

Substitute pears for the apples for
Pear Crumble.

*Calories:* **349** | *Total Fat:* **19g**
*Carbohydrate:* **33g** | *Dietary Fiber:* **8g**
*Protein:* **14g**

## HEALTH BENEFITS:

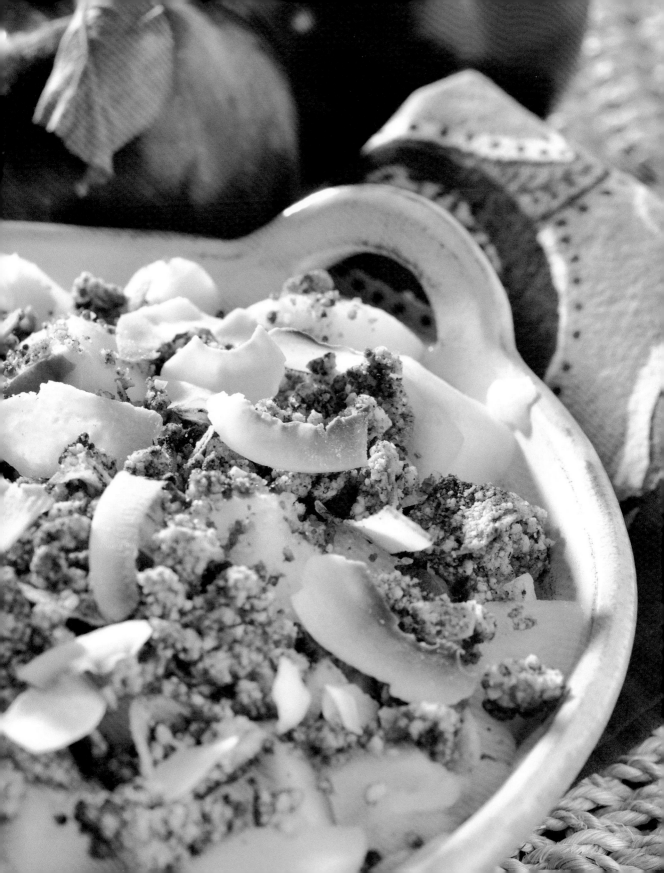

# Almond Butter Balls

*Total time:* **10 minutes** | *Makes* **15 balls**

## INGREDIENTS:

7 tablespoons (14 ounces) Almond Butter (see p. 148)

½ cup almond meal (may ultimately require a bit more depending on the moisture content of the almond butter)

4 tablespoons raw honey (or maple syrup)

## ACTIONS:

1. Combine the Almond Butter, almond meal, and honey (or maple syrup) in a mixing bowl.
2. Roll into balls 1 inch in diameter. You should be able to form the mixture into balls without it sticking to your hands. Add more almond meal, if needed.
3. They are ready to eat! Store the balls in an airtight container in the refrigerator or freezer.

## VARIATIONS:

1. Substitute peanuts for the almonds for Peanut Butter Balls.
2. Substitute Brazil nuts for the almonds for Brazil Nut Balls.
3. Substitute cashews for the almonds for Cashew Nut Balls.
4. Add ½ tablespoon of cacao or more for Chocolate Almond Butter Balls.

*Calories:* **124** | *Total Fat:* **9g**
*Carbohydrate:* **8g** | *Dietary Fiber:* **2g**
*Protein:* **4g**

## HEALTH BENEFITS:

# Raw Cupcakes

*Total time:* **15 minutes preparation, 10 minutes chilling** | *Makes* **8–12 cupcakes**

The cupcakes will stay good in the fridge for 14 days and in the freezer for two months.

## INGREDIENTS:

1 cup walnuts ground into a fine walnut meal

1½ teaspoons pure vanilla extract

1 teaspoon salt

3 tablespoons maple syrup

## ACTIONS:

1. Mix all the ingredients in a bowl. Once well combined, the batter should be slightly moist and moldable. Add water if you need it to be moister.
2. Mold the batter into ½-inch balls and press each one into a paper baking cup.
3. Allow to set in the fridge or freezer for 10 minutes.
4. Ice the cupcakes with Chocolate Sauce (see p. 162) or Chocolate-Avocado Mousse (see p. 168).

## TIPS:

1. Make vanilla icing by mixing coconut butter, maple syrup, and vanilla extract.
2. Make pink icing by adding a few drops of plain beet juice.

## VARIATION:

Add 1 tablespoon cacao powder (or more, if you like a more intense chocolate) to the recipe for Raw Chocolate Cupcakes.

*Calories:* **177** | *Total Fat:* **13g**
*Carbohydrate:* **14g** | *Dietary Fiber:* **2g**
*Protein:* **3g**

## HEALTH BENEFITS:

# Cookie Dough Balls

*Total time:* **15 minutes** | *Makes* **12 balls**

## INGREDIENTS:

**1 cup cashew nuts**
**1 cup gluten-free rolled oats**
**1 teaspoon pure vanilla extract**
**5 teaspoons maple syrup**
**¼ teaspoon salt**
**2 tablespoons cacao nibs**

## ACTIONS:

1. Blend the cashews and oats in a food processor so the mixture resembles the consistency of flour meal. (It should be slightly finer than all-purpose wheat flour.)
2. In a large bowl, combine the nut-oat blend with the vanilla, maple syrup, and salt. Once the mixture is well blended, stir in cacao nibs.
3. Taste. If more moisture is needed, add water; add more maple syrup if you would like the dough to be sweeter.
4. Roll the dough into ½-inch balls and serve.
5. Store uneaten dough balls—if there are any—in the fridge up to three weeks. In the freezer they will stay good for up to two months.

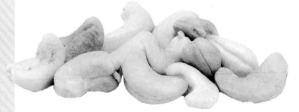

## TIPS:

1. Use vanilla beans if possible. If not, use vanilla extract without added sugar—check the ingredients on the back! If using vanilla beans, scrape the beans from one pod and use them in this recipe.
2. Substitute raw honey for the maple syrup if you prefer.
3. Substitute coconut sugar for the maple syrup if you prefer. Use 3 tablespoons of coconut sugar and 2 tablespoons of water.
4. You can make this recipe without the cacao nibs, however the nibs are what make it like "chocolate chip" cookie dough.
5. These can be made without oats; just use 2 cups of nuts.
6. These are also great made with almonds instead of cashews.

## VARIATIONS:

1. Add 3 tablespoons peanut butter to make Peanut Butter Cookie Dough Balls.
2. On a plate, roll the balls in 1½ tablespoons cacao powder for Chocolate-Covered Cookie Dough Balls.
3. Add 1 tablespoon cacao powder for Chocolate Cookie Dough Balls.
4. Use the crust in the Raw Cherry Pie recipe and fill it with this cookie dough mixture for Cookie Dough Pie.
5. Add a few balls to the Vanilla Smoothie for Cookie Dough Smoothie.

*Calories:* **315** | *Total Fat:* **18g**
*Carbohydrate:* **34g** | *Dietary Fiber:* **4g**
*Protein:* **10g**

## HEALTH BENEFITS:

# Raw Cherry Pie

*Total time:* **20 minutes preparation,**
**additional time to set** | *Makes* **16 slices**

### INGREDIENTS:

*For the pie crust*
**2 cups walnuts**
**2 tablespoons maple syrup or honey**
**1 teaspoon extra-virgin coconut oil**
**¼ teaspoon salt**
**½ teaspoon pure vanilla extract**

*For the filling*
**4 cups pitted cherries**

### ACTIONS:

*For the pie crust*
1. Put the walnuts into a food processor and blend until it forms the consistency of a fine meal (a few chunks of walnut are okay to give it a nice crusty texture).
2. Make the pie crust by adding the walnut meal and other ingredients in a bowl and mix together until it is moist and moldable.
3. Line a pie pan with the pie-crust mixture and press on the bottom as well as the sides until it is even, about ¼-inch thick.

*Putting it together:*
1. Place the cherries in a blender and blend until it is the consistency of a smooth sauce with some chunks, if you like that texture.
2. Pour into the pie crust.
3. Slice and eat right away or set in the refrigerator for 20 minutes. This can also be kept in the freezer as a frozen dessert and will remain fresh for up to 3 months.

### TIPS:
1. Serve with Vegan Ice Cream.
2. If you want a smoother cherry filling, add some coconut oil or maple syrup.
3. For a nut-free version of this pie, use sunflower, pumpkin, or hemp seeds instead of walnuts for the base.
4. You can use 2–3 dates instead of maple syrup in the crust to include more whole foods.
5. Substitute macadamia nuts for the walnuts in the base for a delicious creamy, crunchy pie crust.

### VARIATIONS:
1. To make these square shape, make the recipe in a cake or brownie pan for Walnut Cherry Squares.
2. Substitute pecans for walnuts for Cherry Pecan Pie.
3. Add ¼ cup coconut flakes into the pie crust mixture for Coconut Cherry Pie.
4. Substitute apples for the cherries, following the steps for Apple Pie.
5. Substitute strawberries for the cherries for Strawberry Pie.
6. Add 1 tablespoon of cacao to the pie crust for Chocolate Cherry Pie.

*Calories:* **84** | *Total Fat:* **5g**
*Carbohydrate:* **8g** | *Dietary Fiber:* **2g**
*Protein:* **2g**

### HEALTH BENEFITS:

# Orange Sorbet

*Total time:* **5 minutes** | *Serves* **2**

### INGREDIENTS:

**2 oranges, peeled and seeded**
**4 cups of ice cubes**

### ACTIONS:

1. Place ingredients in a high-speed blender and blend for 1 minute or until you achieve an icy sorbet consistency.
2. Serve immediately.

### TIPS:

1. Add 1–2 tablespoons of honey or maple syrup if you like it sweeter.
2. Add 1 cup of nut milk ice for a creamier sorbet.

### VARIATIONS:

1. Use 2 grapefruits for Grapefruit Sorbet.
2. Use 2 apples for Apple Sorbet.
3. Use 2 peaches for Peach Sorbet.
4. Use 2 cups pineapple chunks for Pineapple Sorbet.
5. Use 2 cups strawberries for Strawberry Sorbet.
6. Use 2 cups passion fruit insides for Passion Fruit Sorbet.
7. Use 2 cups pitted cherries for Cherry Sorbet.
8. Use 2 cups blueberries for Blueberry Sorbet.
9. Use 2 cups raspberries for Raspberry Sorbet.
10. Use ¼ cup each raspberries, blackberries, blueberries, and strawberries for Mixed Berry Sorbet.
11. Grate Chocolate Block (see p. 164) over the orange sorbet for Orange-Chocolate Sorbet.

*Calories:* **62** | *Total Fat:* **0g**
*Carbohydrate:* **15g** | *Dietary Fiber:* **3g**
*Protein:* **1g**

### HEALTH BENEFITS:

WEIGHT LOSS · ENERGY · IMMUNE BOOST · AO · ANTI-INFLAM.

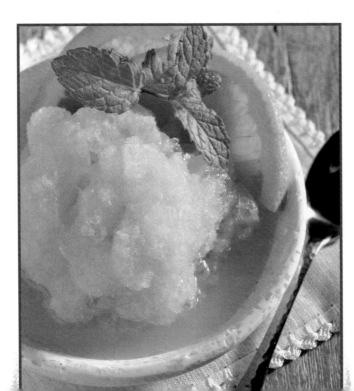

# Vegan Ice Cream

*Total time:* **15 minutes preparation,**
**3–5 hours freezing** | *Serves* **2**

This non-dairy ice cream recipe is wonderful served with fresh fruit, nuts, and/or Chocolate Sauce (see p. 162).

## INGREDIENTS:

**1 cup cashew nuts (substitute sunflower seeds or hemp seeds if you have nut allergies)**
**$^2/_3$ cup Almond Milk (see p. 85) or water**
**1 teaspoon pure vanilla extract**
**4 tablespoons maple syrup**
**$^1/_4$ teaspoon salt**

## ACTIONS:

1. In a food processor, blend all the ingredients until the mixture is as creamy and frothy as you can make it.
2. Pour the mixture into a container. Then, allow the ice cream to set in the freezer for 3–5 hours or overnight.

## TIPS:

1. Using Almond Milk instead of water will give you a creamier ice cream. You can also use Cashew Milk to keep the recipe consistent with only cashews.
2. If you have an ice-cream maker, make the recipe in the blender and then pour it into the ice-cream maker. Allow to churn for 30 minutes to 2 hours in the ice-cream maker until it's ready to eat.
3. The more powerful your blender, the creamier your ice cream will be.
4. Use 1 cup dates instead of maple syrup, if you choose.
5. Soak the cashews for 3 hours for a creamier ice cream.

## VARIATIONS:

1. Add 1 tablespoon (or more, to taste) cacao powder to make Chocolate Ice Cream.
2. Add 1 tablespoon cacao powder and then, after blending, 3 tablespoons cacao nibs to make Chocolate Chip Ice Cream.
3. Add 1 cup strawberries to make Strawberry Ice Cream.
4. Add 1 cup blueberries to make Blueberry Ice Cream.
5. Add 1 tablespoon green tea to make Green Tea Ice Cream.
6. Add 1 tablespoon very finely ground espresso to make Coffee Ice Cream.
7. Drop raw Cookie Dough Balls (see p. 157) into partially frozen ice cream to make Cookie Dough Ice Cream.
8. Add a handful of mint leaves and a drop of mint extract to make Mint Ice Cream.
9. Add a handful of mint leaves, a drop of mint extract, and 1 tablespoon cacao powder to make Chocolate Mint Ice Cream. Add cacao nibs if you want Chocolate Chip Mint Ice Cream.
10. Add the juice of 1–2 lemons for Vanilla-Lemon Ice Cream.
11. Add the juice of 1–2 limes for Vanilla-Lime Ice Cream.
12. Add 1 tablespoon ice cream mixture to paper baking cups for Mini Ice Cream Cakes.

*Calories:* **336** | *Total Fat:* **33g**
*Carbohydrate:* **10g** | *Dietary Fiber:* **2g**
*Protein:* **3g**

## HEALTH BENEFITS:

# Pancakes

*Total time:* **30 minutes** | *Makes* **5–6 pancakes** (5-inch diameter)

### INGREDIENTS:

1 cup rice flour
¹/₂ cup buckwheat flour
³/₄ cup water
1 teaspoon salt
2 tablespoons honey (or maple syrup) plus more for serving
1 egg (vegans can use Flax Egg Alternative recipe as egg replacement [p. 150])
1 teaspoon pure vanilla extract
¹/₄ cup coconut oil for cooking
¹/₂ teaspoon baking soda

### ACTIONS:

1. In a bowl, mix all the ingredients except the coconut oil. Whisk until the batter is well blended and very smooth. Or put all ingredients in a blender.
2. Heat half of the coconut oil in a frying pan. When the oil is hot, pour the batter—about ¹/₄ cup per pancake—into the frying pan.
3. When you see bubbles near the center, flip the pancake.
4. When the pan needs more oil (probably after the third pancake) add remaining oil and continue cooking pancakes.

### TIPS:

1. Serve with fresh fruit like blueberries and strawberries.
2. Serve with maple syrup or honey.
3. Serve with Vegan Ice Cream (see p. 160).
4. Serve with Vegan Butter (see p. 147).
5. Use whole wheat flour if gluten is not an issue for you.

### VARIATIONS:

1. Add an extra ¹/₄ cup water or nut milk to make Crepes.
2. Add 2 tablespoons cacao powder to the batter for Chocolate Pancakes.
3. Add 2 tablespoons of cacao nibs to the batter for Chocolate Chip Pancakes.

*Calories:* **241** | *Total Fat:* **11g**
*Carbohydrate:* **33g** | *Dietary Fiber:* **2g**
*Protein:* **4g**

### HEALTH BENEFITS:

# Freezer Pops

To make flavored freezer pops, use any juice, milkshake, or smoothie recipes in this book. Simply pour them into ice-pop trays, ice trays, or ice molds. Freeze for a few hours and enjoy.

### VARIATIONS:

1. Orange Freezer Pops (see p. 80).
2. Apple Freezer Pops (see p. 80).
3. Slushy Freezer Pops (see p. 94).
4. Chocolate Milk Freezer Pops (see p. 85).
5. Strawberry Smoothie Freezer Pops (see p. 92).
6. Fat Blaster Freezer Pops (see p. 80).

### HEALTH BENEFITS:

> "**Chocolate is an important part of our lives, and now we are learning that it can also provide our body with excellent nutrition.**"
>
> — Noah Loin, Raw Chocolate Man

# Chocolate Sauce

*Total time:* **5 minutes** | *Makes* **1½ cups, serves 6**

Serve as a dip for strawberries and other fruits. Chocolate Sauce also makes a great topping for Vegan Ice Cream.

### INGREDIENTS:

⅔ cup cacao powder
½ cup maple syrup
¼ cup extra-virgin coconut oil

### ACTION:

In a blender, blend all ingredients on high speed until they become a smooth sauce.

### TIPS:

1. For a more intense chocolate flavor, add more cacao powder.
2. For a sweeter flavor, add more maple syrup.
3. If you want the recipe to be raw, substitute raw honey for maple syrup.
4. You can also make this without a blender. Use a bowl and a spoon.

*Calories:* **170** | *Total Fat:* **11g**
*Carbohydrate:* **22g** | *Dietary Fiber:* **3g**
*Protein:* **2g**

### HEALTH BENEFITS:

# Raw Three-ingredient Chocolate

*Total time:* **5 minutes** | *Makes* **1½ cups of chocolate, serves 8**

Making healthy chocolate is easier than you may think. This is one of the most popular recipes I offer. This chocolate can stay fresh in the fridge for 14 days and in the freezer for three months.

### INGREDIENTS:

1 cup nut meal (finely ground almonds or other nut)
¼ cup cacao powder
3 tablespoons maple syrup or raw honey

### ACTIONS:

1. Mix the nut meal, cacao powder, and maple syrup in a bowl.
2. With this mixture, you can roll balls, make squares for brownies, or create a base for a dessert pie!

### TIP:

Add ¼ teaspoon salt and ¼ teaspoon pure vanilla extract for enhanced flavor.

*Calories:* **106** | *Total Fat:* **7g**
*Carbohydrate:* **13g** | *Dietary Fiber:* **4g**
*Protein:* **4g**

### HEALTH BENEFITS:

# Raw Chocolate Balls

*Total time:* **10 minutes** | *Makes* **12 balls**

### INGREDIENTS:

**1 Raw Three-ingredient Chocolate
(see p. 162)**

### ACTION:

Roll the Three-ingredient Chocolate into balls ½-inch in size, and they will be ready to eat.

### VARIATIONS:

1. Add ¼ cup melted cacao butter (the balls will set harder) for Hard Chocolate Balls.
2. Add ¼ teaspoon pure vanilla extract for Chocolate-Vanilla Balls.
3. Add ¼ teaspoon salt for Salty Chocolate Balls.
4. Add 1 drop essential mint oil for Chocolate-Mint Balls.
5. Add 1 tablespoon coconut oil, then roll balls in coconut flakes for Chocolate-Coconut Balls.
6. Add 1 tablespoon peanut butter, and roll into balls for Chocolate Peanut Butter Balls.
7. Add 1 tablespoon Almond Butter (see p. 148) and roll into balls for Chocolate–Almond Butter Balls.
8. Substitute sunflower seeds for nuts to make nut-free Chocolate Sunflower Balls.
9. For High Protein Chocolate Balls, use pumpkin seeds or hemp seeds.

*Calories:* **69** | *Total fat:* **4g**
*Carbohydrate:* **8g** | *Dietary Fiber:* **3g**
*Protein:* **3g**

### HEALTH BENEFITS:

WEIGHT LOSS · ENERGY · DH · AO · IMMUNE BOOST

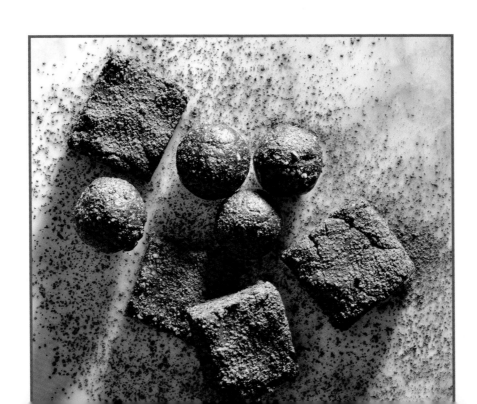

# Chocolate Block

*Total time:* **1 hour** | *Makes* **1 block, serves 8**

### INGREDIENTS:

1 cup cacao butter, unmelted

3 tablespoons raw honey or maple syrup

2 tablespoons cacao powder

1 cup almond meal (or hemp seeds blended into a powdered form)

### ACTIONS:

1. Melt the cacao butter either in the sun or over very low heat on the stove.
2. In a bowl, blend the melted cacao butter, cacao powder, and honey, stirring well so the mixture is thoroughly blended.
3. Add the almond meal to the bowl and stir well again. The result should be smooth.
4. Pour the mixture into chocolate molds or a baking dish, then let set in the freezer or fridge until hard.

### TIPS:

1. The finer the almond meal, the smoother the chocolate will be.
2. To get all of the cacao butter out of the saucepan, add a tablespoon of almond meal and stir it around to soak up the cacao butter.
3. Bonus to working with this ingredient: cacao butter makes a great skin moisturizer!

### VARIATIONS:

1. Add whole nuts to make Chocolate Nut Block.
2. Add raisins, blueberries, and sultanas to make Chocolate Fruit Block.
3. Add fruit and nuts to make Chocolate Fruit Nut Block.
4. For Chocolate Almond Block, add 3 tablespoons almond butter, which will make a creamier chocolate.

*Calories:* **336** | *Total Fat:* **33g**
*Carbohydrate:* **10g** | *Dietary Fiber:* **2g**
*Protein:* **3g**

### HEALTH BENEFITS:

# Raw Chocolate Brownies

*Total time:* **20 minutes** | *Makes* **8 brownies**

### INGREDIENTS:

1 Raw Three-ingredient Chocolate (see p. 162)

### ACTIONS:

1. Pat the mixture into a brownie pan and let set in the fridge for ten minutes.
2. Cut into squares and serve.

### TIPS:

1. Add ¼ teaspoon pure vanilla extract.
2. Add ¼ teaspoon salt.

### VARIATIONS:

1. Ice the brownies with Chocolate-Avocado Mousse (see p. 168) for Iced Chocolate Brownies.
2. Sprinkle coconut flakes on the brownies for Chocolate Coconut Brownies.
3. Add a layer of peanut butter for Chocolate–Peanut Butter Brownies.

*Calories:* **106** | *Total Fat:* **7g**
*Carbohydrate:* **13g** | *Dietary Fiber:* **4g**
*Protein:* **4g**

### HEALTH BENEFITS:

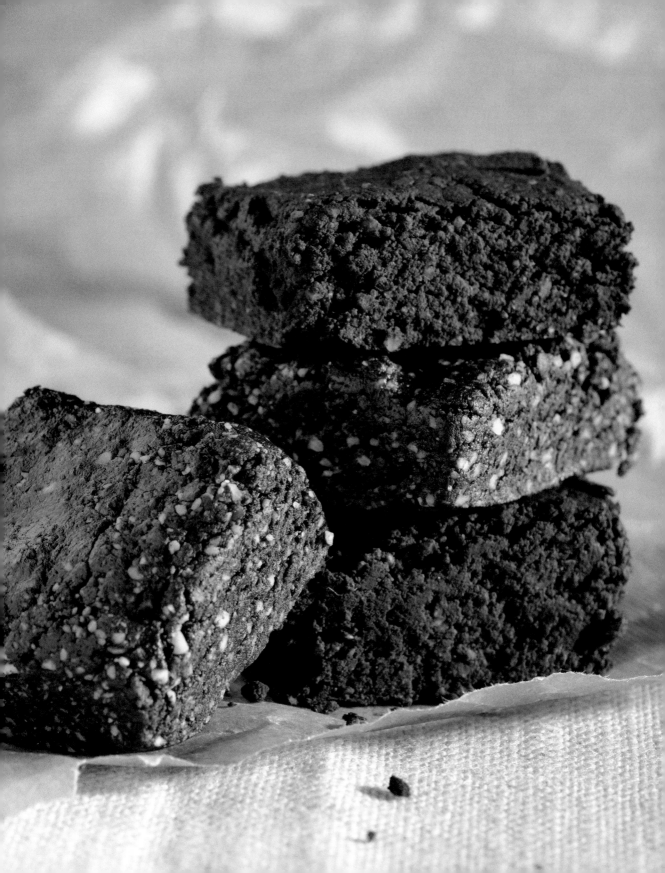

# Raw Chocolate Almond Butter Pie

*Total time:* **20 minutes preparation,**
**2 hours and 20 minutes setting time**
*Makes* **16 slices**

## INGREDIENTS:

*For the base*
½ cup cacao butter
2 tablespoons cacao powder
2 tablespoons maple syrup
¼ cup almond meal
1 tablespoon extra-virgin coconut oil

*For the filling*
14-ounce jar almond butter or 2 cups
of Almond Butter (see p. 148)

*For the icing*
1 avocado
2 tablespoons cacao powder
2 tablespoons maple syrup

## ACTIONS:

*For the base*
1. Melt the cacao butter in the sun or over very low heat on the stove.
2. Once melted, remove from heat, add the remaining base ingredients and mix them well with a spoon.
3. Grease a pie plate with coconut oil, or line a baking sheet with nonstick paper. Pour the base mixture into the pie plate and tilt until the mixture looks flat and smooth.
4. Place the pie plate in the freezer to set until the mixture is hard, approximately 20 minutes.

*For the icing*
1. In a bowl, mash the avocado into a puree.
2. Add the cacao powder and maple syrup and mix until smooth and creamy.

*Putting it together*
1. Remove the pie plate from the freezer.
2. Smooth a layer of almond butter over the chocolate base.
3. Spread the icing over the almond-butter layer.
4. Set in the fridge for two hours and cut into 16 pieces.

## TIPS:

1. For a vanilla base, use this recipe and leave out the cacao powder!
2. For a nut-free version of this pie, use sunflower seeds or hemp seeds whenever it calls for nuts.

## VARIATIONS:

1. Substitute peanut butter for almond butter for Chocolate Peanut Butter Pie.
2. Substitute sunflower butter for almond butter for Chocolate Sunflower Pie.
3. Substitute pumpkin seeds for Chocolate Pumpkin Pie.

*Calories:* **261** | *Total Fat:* **24g**
*Carbohydrate:* **11g** | *Dietary Fiber:* **2g**
*Protein:* **5g**

## HEALTH BENEFITS:

# Flourless Chocolate Cake

*Total making time:* **45 minutes** | *Serves* **12**

## INGREDIENTS:

¼ cup extra-virgin coconut oil
   and more for oiling pan
½ cup (4 ounces) cacao butter
6 tablespoons cacao powder
1 cup coconut sugar
4 eggs, separated

## ACTIONS:

1. Preheat the oven to 350°F.
2. Grease a cake pan with coconut oil.
3. Melt the cacao butter, coconut oil, and cacao powder in a double boiler over simmering water, and mix until smooth. Remove from heat and allow to cool slightly.
4. In a separate bowl, use a hand mixer to beat the egg whites until stiff peaks form. Set aside.
5. In a stand mixer, beat together the coconut sugar and egg yolks until thick and creamy. Mix ¼ of the chocolate mixture into the egg yolks. Continue to mix and slowly pour the remaining chocolate mixture until completely incorporated.
6. Fold the egg whites into the chocolate mixture and mix well.
7. Spoon cake batter into the cake pan.
8. Bake for 25–30 minutes, until the top of the cake begins to crack. Remove from oven and let cool.
9. Garnish with fresh berries or Vegan Ice Cream (see p. 160), or with Chocolate Sauce (see p. 162).

## VARIATIONS:

1. To make Flourless Chocolate Cupcakes, spoon the batter into twelve 4-ounce oven-safe jars to bake, or use a cupcake pan.
2. To make Vegan Flourless Chocolate Cake, use the Flax Egg Alternative (see p. 150) instead of eggs, and then, in Step 4, beat the Flax Egg Alternative until stiff. Continue with Step 5 by adding the coconut sugar and the chocolate mix, and skip Step 6.
3. For Flourless Chocolate Beet Cake, add ½ cup grated raw beet after Step 6. Mix well, pour into cake pan, and bake.

*Calories:* **340** | *Total Fat:* **18g**
*Carbohydrate:* **36g** | *Dietary Fiber:* **2g**
*Protein:* **6g**

## HEALTH BENEFITS:

 ENERGY  AO  DH  ANTI-INFLAM.

# Chocolate-Avocado Mousse

*Total time:* **5 minutes** | *Serves* **1**

## INGREDIENTS:

**1 avocado**

**2 tablespoons cacao powder**

**2 tablespoons raw honey or maple syrup**

## ACTIONS:

1. Blend all ingredients in a food processor until smooth and creamy. (You can also mash the avocado with a fork in a bowl, then add the cacao powder and honey [or maple syrup].)

2. Taste. Add more cacao if you want it more chocolaty. Add more honey if you want it sweeter.

## TIPS:

1. Serve this with fresh raspberries or strawberries!

2. Add ¼ teaspoon pure vanilla extract for enhanced flavor.

3. Add more cacao if you want a richer chocolate and more honey or maple syrup for a sweeter mousse.

4. This is great served on top of ice cream or cupcakes.

*Calories:* **379** | *Total Fat:* **22g**
*Carbohydrate:* **52g** | *Dietary Fiber:* **13g**
*Protein:* **5g**

## HEALTH BENEFITS:

AO · WEIGHT LOSS · ENERGY · DH · IMMUNE BOOST

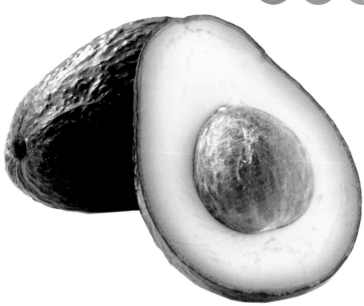

# Chocolate Peanut Butter Cups

*Total time:* **35 minutes** | *Makes* **13 peanut butter cups**

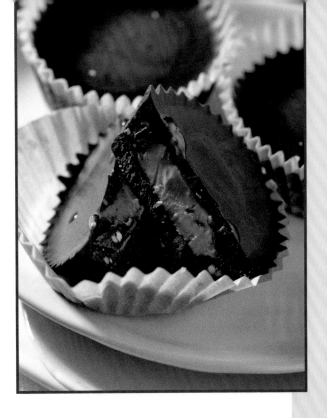

### INGREDIENTS:

3/4 cup cacao butter

3 tablespoons cacao powder

1/2 cup almond meal

3 tablespoons maple syrup

13 teaspoons peanut butter
   (just over 1/4 cup)

13 mini-sized paper baking cups
   (1 5/8-inch diameter)

### ACTIONS:

1. Melt the cacao butter in the sun or over very low heat on the stove. Once melted, add the cacao powder, almond meal, and maple syrup, mixing well. Taste, and then add more cacao if you prefer richer chocolate, and more maple syrup if you prefer a sweeter taste.

2. Spoon 1 teaspoon of the chocolate mixture into the baking cups, filling one-third of the way. Reserve the other half of the mixture for the top of the cups.

3. Put the baking cups in the freezer for 5 minutes to set.

4. Remove the cups from the freezer and add 1 teaspoon peanut butter to each one. Each cup should now be two-thirds full.

5. Add 1 1/2 teaspoons of the remainder of the chocolate mixture into the baking cups.

6. Place the cups in the freezer again, and allow to set for 15 minutes.

### TIPS:

1. Use your favorite nut butter.
2. Add salt to the nut butter, to taste.

### VARIATIONS:

1. Substitute almonds for peanuts for Chocolate Almond Butter Cups.

2. Substitute sunflower seeds for the peanuts and almond meal for nut-free Chocolate Sunflower Cups.

*Calories:* **176** | *Total Fat:* **17g**
*Carbohydrate:* **6g** | *Dietary Fiber:* **1g**
*Protein:* **2g**

### HEALTH BENEFITS:

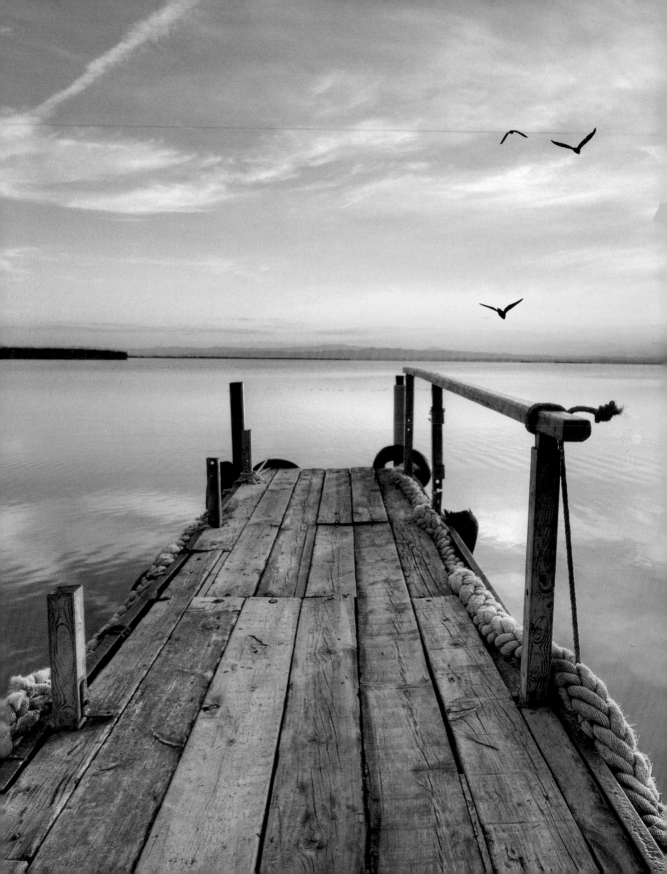

# PART III

# The Earth Diet Guides

"What lies behind us and what
lies before us are tiny matters
compared to what lies within us."
— Ralph Waldo Emerson

# CHAPTER 16

# Weight Loss

## "The most important weight we should shed is the weight of our worries."

— Stephanie Gunning

Losing weight can often simply be a matter of replacing all processed foods with natural, organic foods. If you substitute a healthy ingredient for a processed ingredient, your body will gradually arrive at your ideal weight. It is actually almost inevitable that if you eat healthy foods, with exercise, you will experience living in your dream body in this lifetime. Obsessing about being skinny doesn't work. Jillian Michaels, TV's toughest trainer, said in her book *Master Your Metabolism*, "In my quest to be 'skinny,' I have abused my body for years and years. Rather than getting thinner, I'd succeeded only in aging myself, screwing up my hormone levels, and teaching my body to be *fatter*."

Once I started the Earth Diet, excess weight dropped off me effortlessly. It is such a relief to not be obsessed with my weight anymore. Weight loss requires us to eat nourishing foods and to feel good about ourselves. Kathy Freston is another woman who gets it, and in her book *The Lean*, she says, "Weight loss doesn't require that you put yourself through physical drudgery and live in a constant state of longing or deprivation. That would not make a pleasant life, and no wonder so many of us reject, or fall down on, that hard-core path." Weight loss does not have to be complicated or drive us crazy.

If you desire to accelerate the process, there are a few steps you can take to promote weight loss, such as juicing more frequently. The following Earth Diet recipes have been proven to be powerful for aiding weight loss.

*Warning:* Consult with a doctor before beginning a new diet and if you experience any problems while using these guidelines.

## Top 5 Foods for Weight Loss

1. Beets
2. Kale
3. Cucumber
4. Lemon
5. Grapefruit

## Top 15 Recipes for Weight Loss

1. Beet Juice
2. Green Juice
3. Fat Blaster
4. Weight Loss Tea
5. Lemon Water
6. Coconut Water
7. Ginger Tea
8. Green Salad / Four-ingredient Green Salad
9. Superfood Kale Salad
10. Guacamole
11. Milkshakes (Chocolate, Strawberry, and Vanilla)
12. Smoothies (Chocolate, Banana, and Strawberry)
13. Chocolate Balls
14. Cumin Quinoa
15. Turmeric Rice

# The 15 Most Successful Tips for Weight Loss

1. Follow the Weight Loss Seven-Day Recipe Plan, and implement it periodically for the rest of your life to maintain your ideal weight.
2. Replace all processed foods with recipes from *The Earth Diet*.
3. Cut out all refined sugars.
4. Eat nutrient-rich foods. Nutrition in, cravings out.
5. Juice daily for cellular nutrition.
6. Eat a lot of greens.
7. Eat a majority of raw, living foods.
8. Drink Lemon Water daily to alkalize your body.
9. Reduce stress, by practicing affirmations, positive thinking, and relaxing.
10. Remove gluten from diet.
11. Remove dairy and soy from diet.
12. Breathe and perspire. Jump on a mini-trampoline/rebounder every morning for ten minutes to stimulate your lymphatic system.
13. Eat less or no meat.
14. Eat mono meals, or as simply as possible.
15. Take a hot Epsom salts bath once a week.

# Weight Loss Seven-Day Recipe Plan

**DAY 1**: Lemon Water, Beet Juice, Superfood Kale Salad, Choice of Smoothie, Weight Loss Tea

**DAY 2**: Lemon Water, Green Juice, Superfood Kale Salad, Choice of Smoothie, Weight Loss Tea

**DAY 3**: Lemon Water, Fat Blaster, Superfood Kale Salad, Choice of Smoothie, Weight Loss Tea

**DAY 4**: Lemon Water, Beet Juice, Superfood Kale Salad, Choice of Smoothie, Weight Loss Tea

**DAY 5**: Lemon Water, Green Juice, Superfood Kale Salad, Choice of Smoothie, Weight Loss Tea

**DAY 6**: Lemon Water, Fat Blaster, Superfood Kale Salad, Choice of Smoothie, Weight Loss Tea

**DAY 7**: Lemon Water, Beet Juice, Superfood Kale Salad, Choice of Smoothie, Weight Loss Tea

You may replace any of the recipes in this menu with another recipe for weight loss. For example, you might replace the Superfood Kale Salad with a Green Salad.

If you are craving chocolate during the seven days of this plan, make the Chocolate Balls. And if you still feel hungry after consuming everything that's already on the plan for the day, go ahead and eat a piece of raw fruit, a serving of Guacamole, or a Chocolate Ball.

# Weight Loss Super Acceleration Strategy: Eating Mono Meals for One Day of the Week

**AFTER WAKING**: Lemon Water

**BREAKFAST**: Beet Juice

**NEXT MEAL**: Bananas, until you are full

**LUNCH**: Watermelon, until you are full

**NEXT MEAL**: Grapes, until you are full

**DINNER**: Raw cauliflower, until you are full

**BEFORE BED**: Ginger Tea

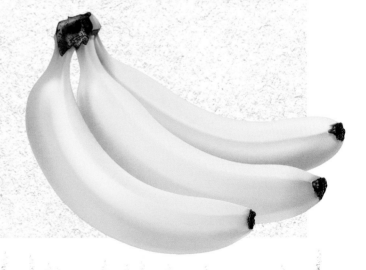

# CHAPTER 17

# Clear Skin

## "For attractive lips, speak words of kindness."

— Sam Levenson (Audrey Hepburn cited this advice as part of her beauty regimen)

To detoxify and rejuvenate your skin, and maintain clear skin, simply replace processed foods and sugars in your diet with natural, organic foods. Use the Earth Diet recipes, which means you will not be consuming dairy, gluten, or soy; and juice daily.

My readers have told me how the following recipes, in particular, have helped them maintain clear, healthy skin and heal from acne, psoriasis, eczema, warts, and other skin conditions.

In addition to changing your diet, you can nourish your skin by topically applying avocado, coconut oil, the interior of aloe vera leaves, and cucumber to it. You may experience a flare-up before it clears up.

*Warning:* Consult with a doctor before beginning a new diet and if you experience any problems while following these guidelines.

## Top 5 Foods for Clear Skin

1. Beets
2. Cucumber
3. Celery
4. Lemon
5. Kale

## Top 15 Recipes for Clear Skin

1. Beet Juice
2. Green Juice
3. Lemon Water
4. Superfood Kale Salad
5. Green Salad / Four-ingredient Salad
6. Fat Blaster
7. Orange Juice
8. Ginger Tea
9. Coconut Water
10. Coconut Milk
11. Guacamole
12. Smoothies (Chocolate, Banana, and Strawberry)
13. Chocolate Balls
14. Cumin Quinoa
15. Turmeric Rice

# The 15 Most Successful Tips for Clear Skin

1. Follow the Clear Skin Recipe Plan for seven days—and after that you may implement it whenever you get a flare-up.

2. Nutrition in, toxins out. Replace all processed foods with recipes from *The Earth Diet*.

3. Juice daily for instant cellular nutrition.

4. If you have intense acne, psoriasis, eczema, warts, or other skin issues, you can do a juice detox with the Seven-Day Juice Cleanse to give your organs a deep flush-out of toxins.

5. For moisturizing, use organic extra-virgin coconut oil. For a lush moisturizer, mix ¾ cup extra-virgin olive oil, 1 tablespoon raw honey, and 1 tablespoon chamomile flowers (either loose leaf or taken from a tea bag) in a high-speed blender. Apply to skin and massage.

6. For anti-aging and to reduce redness and inflammation, apply aloe or cucumber slices to your skin, wait 20 minutes, then wash.

7. Apple cider vinegar, diluted with an equal measure of water, acts as a skin toner.

8. Eat a majority of raw, living foods.

9. Only use organic, natural skin-care products. Make sure there are no harsh, toxic chemical ingredients.

10. Drink Lemon Water daily to alkalize your body.

11. Use bentonite clay for a face mask that reduces the appearance of wrinkles. (This is nature's version of Botox.) When you purchase the clay, the directions are on the package.

12. For an antioxidant cacao face mask, mix ¼ cup organic extra-virgin coconut oil with 1 tablespoon cacao powder. Apply to your skin and leave on for 20 minutes before rinsing thoroughly.

13. Remember: If you can't eat it, do not put it on your skin!

14. Eat mono meals, or as simply as possible.

15. Mash up an avocado and smooth it onto your face. Let it set for 15 minutes, then wash off.

# Clear Skin Seven-Day Recipe Plan

**DAY 1:** Lemon Water, Beet Juice, Superfood Kale Salad, 3 celery sticks, Choice of Smoothie, Ginger Tea

**DAY 2:** Lemon Water, Green Juice, Four-ingredient Green Salad, cucumber, Choice of Smoothie, Ginger Tea

**DAY 3:** Lemon Water, Orange Juice, Superfood Kale Salad, Guacamole, Choice of Smoothie, Ginger Tea

**DAY 4:** Lemon Water, Beet Juice, Four-ingredient Green Salad, Choice of Smoothie, cucumber, Ginger Tea

**DAY 5:** Lemon Water, Green Juice, Superfood Kale Salad, cucumber, Choice of Smoothie, Ginger Tea

**DAY 6:** Lemon Water, Fat Blaster, Four-ingredient Green Salad, Guacamole, Choice of Smoothie, Ginger Tea

**DAY 7:** Lemon Water, Beet Juice, Superfood Kale Salad, cucumber, Choice of Smoothie, Ginger Tea

**SNACKS:** Coconut Water, Chocolate Balls, Freezer Pops, cucumber, celery sticks

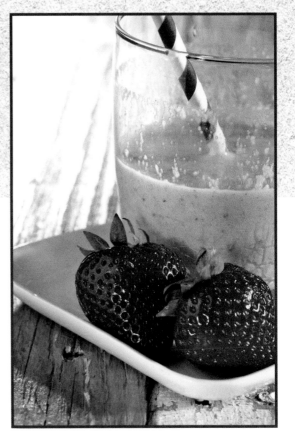

# CHAPTER 18

# Eating Desserts Daily

## We are living in great times, a time when we can have our cake and eat it, too!

To be able to eat dessert every day, simply replace all the processed desserts in your diet with natural, organic desserts. Use the Earth Diet dessert recipes. The following recipes in particular will help you be successful in maintaining a healthy lifestyle and keep your energy high, while also being decadently delicious, fulfilling, and easy to make. These desserts are happy foods, as they release serotonin in the brain and excite the body. A happy body is a healthy body! Not only are these desserts packed with nutrition, they also taste like typical desserts. This guide can be helpful for people who are addicted to junk-food desserts and want to break the addiction by replacing all those cravings with these natural desserts. When you crave chocolate, make Raw Chocolate Balls, and when you crave ice cream, eat Vegan Ice Cream.

*Warning:* Consult with a doctor before beginning a new diet and if you experience any problems while following these guidelines.

### 15 Guilt-free Desserts You Could Eat Daily

1. Raw Chocolate Balls
2. Chocolate Brownies
3. Chocolate Block
4. Raw Cashew Cheesecake
5. Ice Cream
6. Freezer Pops
7. Cookie Dough Balls
8. Raw Chocolate Almond Butter Pie
9. Raw Cupcakes
10. Pancakes
11. Almond Butter Balls
12. Apple Crumble
13. Chocolate Mousse
14. Chocolate Smoothie
15. Strawberry Milkshake

# 10 Tips for
# Eating Desserts Daily

1. Follow the Eating Desserts Seven-Day Recipe Plan (below).

2. Replace refined sugars with natural sugars like dates, raw honey, and maple syrup.

3. Eat a majority of raw, rather than cooked, desserts. Raw desserts are also vegan and plant-based, which means they're easier for the body to digest and won't cause weight gain.

4. Eat gluten-free desserts. (All Earth Diet desserts are gluten free!)

5. Eat dairy-free desserts. (All Earth Diet desserts are dairy free!)

6. Eat soy-free desserts. (All Earth Diet desserts are soy free!)

7. Eat desserts made with organic ingredients.

8. Eat desserts made with non-GMO ingredients.

9. Eat desserts that flood your body with nutrients, as well as taste really good.

10. Eat desserts free of chemicals, preservatives, colorings, additives, and other toxic ingredients.

# Eating Desserts Seven-Day Recipe Plan

**DAY 1:** Lemon Water, Beet Juice, 2–3 Chocolate Balls, Superfood Kale Salad, a handful of Chocolate Block, Mixed Berry Smoothie, Turmeric Rice, Cheesecake, Ginger Tea

**DAY 2:** Lemon Water, Green Juice, Cheesecake, Superfood Kale Salad, 2–3 Chocolate Balls, Strawberry Smoothie, Cumin Quinoa, Chocolate Block, Ginger Tea

**DAY 3:** Lemon Water, Fat Blaster, Chocolate Block, Turmeric Rice, Cheesecake, Chocolate Smoothie, Superfood Kale Salad, 2–3 Chocolate Balls, Ginger Tea

**DAY 4:** Lemon Water, Beet Juice, 2–3 Chocolate Balls, Cumin Quinoa, a handful of Chocolate Block, Strawberry Milkshake, Superfood Kale Salad, Cheesecake, Ginger Tea

**DAY 5:** Lemon Water, Green Juice, Cheesecake, Chocolate Smoothie, Superfood Kale Salad, a handful of Chocolate Block, Turmeric Rice, 2–3 Chocolate Balls, Ginger Tea

**DAY 6:** Lemon Water, Fat Blaster, a handful of Chocolate Block, Superfood Kale Salad, Mixed Berry Smoothie, Cheesecake, Cumin Quinoa, 2–3 Chocolate Balls, Ginger Tea

**DAY 7:** Lemon Water, Beet Juice, 2–3 Chocolate Balls, Turmeric Rice, Strawberry Smoothie, a handful of Chocolate Block, Superfood Kale Salad, Cheesecake, Ginger Tea

**SNACKS:** avocado and cucumber

# Design Your Own Once-a-Week "Day of Desserts" Plan

Pick one day of the week on which to make three of your favorite dessert recipes from *The Earth Diet*. (*The Earth Diet* desserts will stay fresh in the fridge for 7–14 days and the freezer 14–90 days, if stored in an airtight container.) Let's say, for instance, that you choose to make the Chocolate Balls, Chocolate Block, and Cheesecake. Your days will look like this:

**AFTER WAKING:** Lemon Water

**BREAKFAST:** Choice of Juice

**NEXT MEAL:** Choice of Dessert (perhaps Cheesecake?)

**LUNCH:** Superfood Kale Salad and Choice of Dessert (perhaps a handful of Chocolate Block?)

**NEXT MEAL:** Choice of Smoothie

**DINNER:** Turmeric Rice and Choice of Dessert (perhaps Raw Chocolate Balls?)

**BEFORE BED:** Herbal Tea

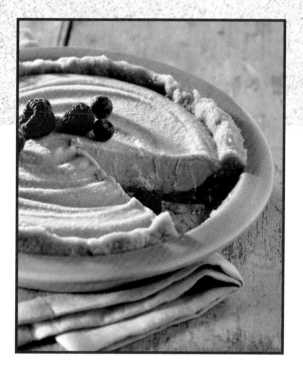

# CHAPTER 19

# High Protein

### "I'm a huge believer in the idea that when you start the week off right, you're more likely to end it better as well."

— Curtis Stone

To gain weight and build muscle naturally, replace all processed foods in your diet with natural, organic foods that are high in protein. Use the Earth Diet recipes in this book. The following recipes are particularly useful for people who want to build and tone muscle, want to gain weight, and need assistance in recovering after their workouts. These are great sources of protein both for athletes and people who require more protein and energy. You can simply add more protein to your foods by adding Protein Powder (see p. 104) to your smoothies, salads, soups, and cereals.

*Warning:* Consult with a doctor before beginning a new diet and if you experience any problems while following these guidelines.

## Top 5 High-Protein Foods for Meat Eaters

1. Chicken
2. Red meat
3. Fish
4. Shrimp
5. Eggs

## Top 12 High-Protein Recipes for Meat Eaters

1. Roast Chicken
2. Chicken Nuggets
3. Honey Rosemary Chicken
4. Burgers
5. Fish and Chips
6. Simple Sage Fish
7. Beef Stir-Fry
8. Caramel Shrimp
9. Beef Burritos
10. Baked Crusted Salmon
11. Baked Lamb Chops
12. Omelet

# Meat Eaters' Seven-Day High-Protein Recipe Plan

**DAY 1:** Lemon Water, Beet Juice, Banana Smoothie, Breakfast Cereal, Egg Omelet, Chocolate Brownie, Chicken Nuggets, Superfood Kale Salad

**DAY 2:** Lemon Water, Green Juice, Banana Smoothie, Breakfast Cereal, Egg Omelet, Chocolate Brownie, Honey-Rosemary Chicken, Superfood Kale Salad

**DAY 3:** Lemon Water, Orange Juice, Banana Smoothie, Breakfast Cereal, Egg Omelet, Chocolate Brownie, Beef Stir-Fry, Superfood Kale Salad

**DAY 4:** Lemon Water, Beet Juice, Banana Smoothie, Breakfast Cereal, Egg Omelet, Chocolate Brownie, Fish and Chips, Superfood Kale Salad

**DAY 5:** Lemon Water, Green Juice, Banana Smoothie, Breakfast Cereal, Egg Omelet, Chocolate Brownie, Burgers, Superfood Kale Salad

**DAY 6:** Lemon Water, Orange Juice, Banana Smoothie, Breakfast Cereal, Egg Omelet, Chocolate Brownie, Caramel Shrimp, Superfood Kale Salad

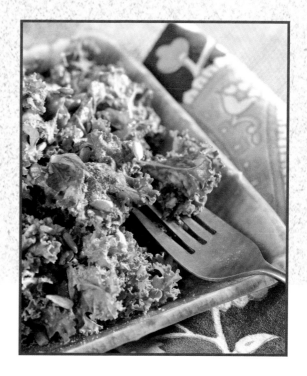

**DAY 7:** Lemon Water, Beet Juice, Banana Smoothie, Breakfast Cereal, Egg Omelet, Chocolate Brownie, Roast Chicken, Superfood Kale Salad

**SNACKS:** Raw nuts, Smoothie, Chocolate Brownie, Guacamole, hemp seeds, pumpkin seeds

**TIP:** Swap any of the recipes with the other top high-protein recipes.

## Top 10 High-Protein Foods for Vegans

1. Hemp seeds
2. Pumpkin seeds
3. Peanuts
4. Almonds
5. Lentils
6. Quinoa
7. Kale
8. Chickpeas
9. Beans
10. Rice

## Top 15 High-Protein Recipes for Vegans

1. Superfood Kale Salad
2. Protein Powder
3. Lentil Soup
4. Almond Butter, Peanut Butter, Pumpkin Seed Butter
5. Hummus
6. Mac 'n' Cheese
7. Raw Pizza
8. Cumin Quinoa
9. Vegan Curry
10. Bean Burgers
11. Zucchini Pasta with Pesto
12. Raw Tacos
13. Zucchini Pasta with Walnut Meat Balls
14. Raw Lasagna
15. Breakfast Cereal

# Vegan Seven-Day High-Protein Recipe Plan

**DAY 1:** Lemon Water, Beet Juice, Banana Smoothie, Breakfast Cereal, Chocolate Brownie, Superfood Kale Salad, Turmeric Rice

**DAY 2:** Lemon Water, Green Juice, Banana Smoothie, Breakfast Cereal, Chocolate Brownie, Cumin Quinoa, Superfood Kale Salad

**DAY 3:** Lemon Water, Orange Juice, Banana Smoothie, Breakfast Cereal, Chocolate Brownie, Superfood Kale Salad, Mac 'n' Cheese

**DAY 4:** Lemon Water, Beet Juice, Banana Smoothie, Breakfast Cereal, Bean Burgers, Chocolate Brownie, Superfood Kale Salad, Lentil Soup

**DAY 5:** Lemon Water, Green Juice, Banana Smoothie, Breakfast Cereal, Guacamole, Chocolate Brownie, Superfood Kale Salad, Raw Lasagna

**DAY 6:** Lemon Water, Orange Juice, Banana Smoothie, Breakfast Cereal, Superfood Kale Salad, Chocolate Brownie, Zucchini Pasta and Walnut Meat Balls

**DAY 7:** Lemon Water, Beet Juice, Banana Smoothie, Breakfast Cereal, Chocolate Brownie, Raw Pizza, Superfood Kale Salad

**SNACKS:** Any Smoothie, Chocolate Brownie, raw nuts, Guacamole, pumpkin seeds, hemp seeds, Hummus

**TIPS:** If you don't want a Banana Smoothie, swap it out for a Chocolate, Strawberry, or Mixed Berry Smoothie. For extra protein, add 1 – 3 tablespoons of Almond Butter, Peanut Butter, or Protein Powder to your smoothie.

High Protein

# CHAPTER 20

# Boosting Your Immunity

Follow these guidelines whether your body needs light healing or deep healing. It is helpful for improving relatively simple conditions, ranging from not feeling well and being low in energy or feeling fatigued, to being sick in bed with a head cold, the flu, or a virus. Readers with diverse conditions such as cancer, diabetes, digestive issues, and skin issues have reported that they feel stronger after even a few days of following these guidelines. You can use this plan just because you feel like nourishing your body. It seems like common sense to me that if we boost our immune systems regularly, we are more likely to be able to fight off or overcome any type of sickness.

*Warning:* Consult with a doctor before beginning a new diet and if you experience any problems while following these guidelines.

## Top 5 Immune-boosting Foods

1. Lemon
2. Celery
3. Kale
4. Berries
5. Turmeric

> "Take care of your body. It's the only place you have to live."
>
> — Jim Rohn

## 15 Tips for Boosting Your Immunity

1. Eat only organic produce and meats.

2. Eat a majority of raw, living, whole, organic foods.

3. Drink Immune-boosting Juice (see p. 79).

4. Drink Immune-boosting Tea (see p. 97).

# The Immune-boosting Seven-Day Recipe Plan

The following seven-day menu for boosting your immunity is high in vitamins, minerals, and antioxidants. The plan is based on mostly raw vegan recipes, but includes two cooked healing recipes: Cumin Quinoa and Turmeric Rice. If you are someone who exclusively eats raw vegan style, substitute another Smoothie or Juice of your choice for these two meals in your own personal plan.

**DAY 1:** Lemon Water, Green Juice, Mixed Berry Smoothie, Superfood Kale Salad, Immune-boosting Juice, Cumin Quinoa, Immune-boosting Tea

**DAY 2:** Lemon Water, Immune-boosting Juice, Banana Smoothie, Superfood Kale Salad, Beet Juice, Turmeric Rice, Immune-boosting Tea

**DAY 3:** Lemon Water, Orange Juice, Mixed Berry Smoothie, Superfood Kale Salad, Immune-boosting Juice, Cumin Quinoa, Immune-boosting Tea

**DAY 4:** Lemon Water, Immune-boosting Juice, Chocolate Smoothie, Turmeric Rice, Green Juice, Superfood Kale Salad, Immune-boosting Tea

**DAY 5:** Lemon Water, Orange Juice, Strawberry Smoothie, Cumin Quinoa, Immune-boosting Juice, Superfood Kale Salad, Immune-boosting Tea

**DAY 6:** Lemon Water, Immune-boosting Juice, Mixed Berry Smoothie, Turmeric Rice, Beet Juice, Superfood Kale Salad, Immune-boosting Tea

**DAY 7:** Lemon Water, Green Juice, Chocolate Smoothie, Superfood Kale Salad, Immune-boosting Juice, Turmeric Rice, Immune-boosting Tea

**SNACKS:** celery, cucumber, berries

5. Drink Lemon Water daily for vitamin C and cellular nutrition (see p. 100).

6. Get coffee enemas to stimulate your digestive system. Look for a health-care professional in your area who can do this for you or see the Recommended Resources section on my website for information about home kits.

7. Drink Beet Juice to cleanse your colon (see p. 77).

8. Drink Green Juice to increase your energy (see p. 78).

9. Eat ginger.

10. Eat turmeric.

11. Eat garlic.

12. Drink clean water.

13. Eat alkalizing foods.

14. Drink bentonite clay (see p. 192) to absorb parasites, toxins, and heavy metals.

15. Commit to feeling good. It is essential that we learn to reduce stress and nurture ourselves emotionally so we may feel good the majority of the time. The body is more resilient when we are happy.

# CHAPTER 21

# Seven-Day Juice Cleanse

### "Reboot your life."

— Joe Cross

Feel free to do the juice cleanse whenever you feel like getting a high dose of nutrients and vitamins at a cellular level. The benefits of the Seven-Day Juice Cleanse include losing weight, detoxifying, boosting the immune system, increasing energy, cleansing the body of free radicals and GMOs, flushing the digestive system, clearing the skin, clearing out allergies, and more.

During your cleanse, you may experience detoxification symptoms, such as feeling unwell, drunk, imbalanced, and tired. This is normal, as the body is flushing out toxins. During these times remember the symptoms will pass. Things that can help to get out the toxins while you put nutrition in are sweating in a sauna, light exercise, walking, stretching, and using a dry body brush.

Your mind might tell you that you are not getting all the nutrients you need, but let me assure you, you will be getting more nutrients than usual as the nutrition from the juice is going into your body at the cellular level.

*Warning:* Consult with a doctor before beginning a new diet and if you experience any problems while following these guidelines. Juice cleansing is not recommended for pregnant women, as flushing toxins while growing a baby is not a good idea.

## Top 5 Detoxifying Foods

1. Beet
2. Kale
3. Cucumber
4. Celery
5. Ginger

# Seven-Day Juice Cleanse Instructions

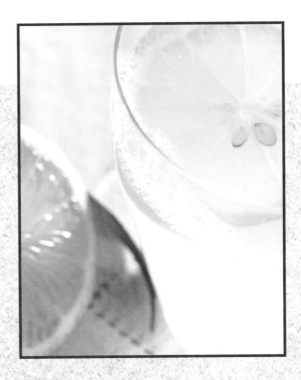

Drink an Earth Diet juice every two hours until your day ends and you go to bed. Repeat for seven days.

**THIS IS THE RECOMMENDED ORDER:**

**UPON WAKING:** Lemon Water

**7 A.M.:** Green Juice

**9 A.M.:** Beet Juice

**11 A.M.:** Apple Cucumber Ginger Juice

**1 P.M.:** Fat Blaster

**3 P.M.:** Immune-boosting Juice

**5 P.M.:** Celery Juice

**7 P.M.:** Vegetable Juice

**BEFORE SLEEPING:** Weight Loss Tea

For accelerated health benefits, some people continue their juice cleanses for 21 days. Watch the film *Fat, Sick, and Nearly Dead* by Joe Cross for inspiration.

# "Look deep into nature, and then you will understand everything better."

— Albert Einstein

At the Earth Diet, we're committed to supporting you in leading a natural, earth-friendly lifestyle. To this end, we have created lifestyle and eating programs catering to your specific needs.

## Earth Diet Health Coaching

Work with myself or another personal health coach to meet your personal dietary and lifestyle goals. We create personalized programs for each individual. For details, visit TheEarthDiet.com.

## Earth Diet Downloadable Programs

You may be interested in our downloadable 7-day, 21-day, 60-day, or 90-day programs for weight loss, nourishment, diabetes, juice cleansing, clear skin, energy, cellulite, fertility, pregnancy, and more. For details, visit TheEarthDiet.com.

## Connect with Me Via Social Networks and On-air

I would love to connect with you after you've read this book. To keep in touch, either e-mail me directly at liana@theearthdiet.org, or join me through my various social media accounts.
**FACEBOOK:** Facebook.com/theearthdiet
**TWITTER:** Twitter.com/theearthdieter
**PINTEREST:** Pinterest.com/theearthdiet
**INSTAGRAM:** Instagram.com/theearthdiet
**YOUTUBE:** Youtube.com/theearthdiet

## Read My Blog, TheEarthDiet.blogspot.com

This is where the Earth Diet started. Fed up with a five-year addiction to junk food and binge eating, I created a challenge for myself to end the vicious cycle by eating only unrefined organic foods for the next 365 days. Now my posts focus on leading a wholesome lifestyle and offering hundreds of delicious and healing recipes I've created that have helped thousands of people around the world.

## Earth Diet Food Demonstrations and Lectures

I frequently travel the world to give cooking demonstrations and food lectures. An appearance might include a demonstration on how to make raw chocolate balls, or some helpful tips for self-healing. To see when I might be coming to a town near you, visit TheEarthDiet.com/tour.

To book me for your event, e-mail: info@theearthdiet.org.

**FOR A FREE GIFT, PLEASE VISIT THEEARTHDIET.COM/BOOKGIFT**

## Earth Diet—Approved Stuff

In the pages that follow, you will find a list of informational products—books, audio programs, films, websites, newsletters—designed to educate you further, as well as a list of credible organizations that can support you in leading an earth-friendly, organic lifestyle. Of course, it is important for you to remember that it is always up to you to use your personal wisdom to identify the choices that are appropriate to assist you in living your own healthiest life.

## Recommended Books

These books are recommended because they can empower each of us to live a healthy, peaceful life and support us in creating a consistent state of well-being.

### FOR THE BODY

*A Course in Weight Loss*
by Marianne Williamson

*Dying to Be Me*
by Anita Moorjani

*Heal Your Body A–Z*
by Louise Hay

*Healthy at 100*
by John Robbins

*Mind Over Medicine*
by Lissa Rankin

*Reinventing the Body*
by Deepak Chopra

*The Biology of Belief*
by Bruce Lipton

*The China Study*
by T. Colin Campbell

*The Four Agreements*
by Don Miguel Ruiz

*The Honeymoon Effect*
by Bruce Lipton

*The Only Answer to Cancer*
by Leonard Coldwell

*The UltraMind Solution*
by Mark Hyman, M.D.

*The Secret Pleasures of Menopause*
by Christiane Northrup, M.D.

### FOR THE MIND AND SPIRIT

*A Return to Love*
by Marianne Williamson

*All Is Well* by Louise Hay

*Buddha's Little Instruction Book*
by Jack Kornfield

*Change Your Thoughts, Change Your Life*
by Wayne Dyer

*Excuses Begone*
by Wayne Dyer

*Happy for No Reason*
by Marci Shimoff

*Long Walk to Freedom*
by Nelson Mandela

*May Cause Miracles*
by Gabrielle Bernstein

*The Power of Now*
by Eckhart Tolle

*When Things Fall Apart*
by Pema Chödrön

*You Can Heal Your Life*
by Louise Hay

### FOR THE EARTH

*A New Earth*
by Eckhart Tolle

*Seeds of Deception*
by Jeffrey Smith

*The Omnivore's Dilemma*
by Michael Pollan

*Second Nature*
by Michael Pollan

*Organic Farming*
by Peter V. Fossel

*The Organic Farming Manual*
by Anne Larkin Hansen

*The Food Revolution*
by John Robbins

### FOR THE HOME

*Organic Housekeeping*
by Ellen Sandbeck

## Recommended Audio Programs

It can be helpful to listen to these inspirational audio programs when in the car, at home, or even in the background as you wash dishes.

*Meditation: Practicing Presence in Every Moment of Your Life*
by Eckhart Tolle

*Meditations for a Miraculous Life*
by Marianne Williamson

*The Importance of Being Extraordinary*
by Wayne Dyer and Eckhart Tolle

*The Wisdom of Your Cells*
by Bruce Lipton

*You Can Heal Your Life Study Course*
by Louise Hay

## Recommended Films

The following documentaries reveal ways to heal using the power of natural foods and expose the dangers of toxic ingredients and hazardous practices within the food industry.

### ON NUTRITIONAL HEALING

*Burzysnki, the Movie—Cancer Is Serious Business*, directed by Eric Merola

*Crazy Sexy Cancer*, directed by Kris Carr

*Fat, Sick and Nearly Dead*, directed by Joe Cross and Kurt Engfehr

*Free Food and Medicine*, directed by Markus Rothkranz

*I Cure Cancer*, directed by Ian Jacklin

*The Gerson Miracle*, directed by Steve Kroschel

*The Joy of Juicing*, directed by Gary Null, Ph.D., and Valerie Van Cleve

### ON THE FOOD INDUSTRY

*Sweet Misery: A Poisoned World*, directed by J. T. Waldron and Cori Brackett

*Food, Inc.*, directed by Robert Kenner

*Food Matters*, directed by James Colquhoun and Laurentine Ten Bosch

*Genetic Roulette*, directed by Jeffrey Smith

*Sugar: The Bitter Truth*, a lecture by Robert H. Lustig, M.D. (available on YouTube.com)

*Super Size Me*, directed by Morgan Spurlock

*The World According to Monsanto*, directed by Marie-Monique Robin

*War on Health*, directed by Gary Null, Ph.D.

## Recommended Websites

The following websites have helped me and many others overcome sickness of mind and body, and to connect with nature and live a positive, organic lifestyle.

DORway.com
For information on aspartame poisoning

FoodRevolution.org
The blog of John Robbins and Ocean Robbins

Honest.com
The website, blog, and tips to building a household with healthy materials from actress and author of *The Honest Life*, Jessica Alba

# Recommended Organizations

## BURZYNSKI CLINIC

Established in 1977, the Burzynski Clinic has grown to a world-renowned cancer center that provides advanced and cutting-edge cancer treatments. The clinic is nationally, as well as internationally, recognized.

9432 Katy Freeway
Houston, Texas 77055
Website: BurzynskiClinic.com
(800) 714-7181 (toll free)

## THE TREE OF LIFE REJUVENATION CENTER

The Tree of Life was founded by Gabriel Cousens, M.D., M.D. (H), to support and inspire holistic lifestyle through education and experience. The center's spiritual guidance, lifestyle education, and medical programs are complemented with panoramic mountain views and 100 percent organic, live-food meals that have drawn guests from over 100 countries since 1995.

686 Harshaw Road
Patagonia, Arizona 85624
Website: GabrielCousens.com
(866) 394-2520 (toll free for United States and Canada)
(520) 233-7010 (international)

## INSTITUTE FOR INTEGRATIVE NUTRITION

Study and get a degree at the Institute for Integrative Nutrition. Its mission is to play a crucial role in improving health and happiness, and through that process, create a ripple effect that transforms the world. To potentially get $1,000 off your tuition and become an Earth Diet health coach, visit TheEarthDiet.com/StudyNutrition.

3 East 28th Street, 12th floor
New York, New York 10016
Website: IntegrativeNutrition.com
(877) 730-5444 (United States)
(212) 730-5433 (international)

## OLIVIA NEWTON-JOHN CANCER AND WELLNESS CENTRE AT THE AUSTIN HOSPITAL

The Olivia Newton-John Cancer & Wellness Centre at the Austin Hospital stands amongst the best in the world, dedicated to providing the very best medical treatment and supportive care for cancer patients and their families. It includes an integrated research facility, to help speed up the process of searching for and implementing new treatments to help stop cancer from spreading and occurring.

145 Studley Road, Heidelberg
Victoria, Australia 3084
Website: Oliviaappeal.com
(03) 9496-5000

## THE GERSON INSTITUTE

The Gerson Institute is a non-profit organization in San Diego, California, dedicated to providing education and training in the Gerson Therapy—an alternative, non-toxic treatment for cancer and other chronic degenerative diseases.

P.O. Box 161358
San Diego, CA 92176
Website: Gerson.org
(888) 443-7766 (toll free for United States and Canada)
(619) 685-5353 (best for international)

## HIPPOCRATES INSTITUTE

Resting among 50 acres of tropical woodlands in southern Florida, Hippocrates offers a serene setting in which to heal, nurture, and develop into one's fullest potential. The institute's signature Life Transformation Program provides fundamental training and a definitive blueprint for transitioning to a healthier lifestyle.

1466 Hippocrates Way
West Palm Beach, FL 33411
(888) 228-1755 (United States)
(561) 471-8876 (international)

## Recommended Purchases

These are the first 7 things I recommend you buy when starting this lifestyle.

1. **VITAMIX:** Use this to make smoothies, juices, nut milk, raw desserts like ice cream and cheesecake, and more. Get a discount using a promo code on my website. Vitamix is known as one of the most reliable blenders in the world.

2. **PHRESH GREENS:** This is an alkaline green drink made from green superfoods formed into an organic greens powder. You can get a complete daily serving of raw greens in 1 teaspoon. This product helps me when I am traveling or on the go and don't have time to make a fresh juice. Get a discount from my website.

3. **BENTONITE CLAY:** Drink ¼ teaspoon daily with water to absorb toxins like GMOs, parasites, worms, heavy metals, and radioactivity. Also aids weight loss and digestive healing. Available on my website.

4. **RAW CHOCOLATE:** Have healthy chocolate with you and in your home, so when you have a craving, you're prepared. I love to eat chocolate every day, so now I have my very own line of Chocolate Peanut Butter Cups and Chocolate Almond Butter Cups. Get them at your local health-food store or shop on my website.

5. **WATER FILTER:** On my website, I recommend different types based on your budget. We should always drink and bathe in clean, chemical-free water.

6. **JUICE MACHINE:** So you can juice everyday! They range from $40 to thousands. You can get a good-quality juice machine for $100.

7. **HIRE YOUR OWN HEALTH COACH:** You can either download a program or hire a health coach so that you have your own personalized, one-on-one coaching. I designed these programs for people who want to take it to the next level and experience transformative results, whether that means moving toward healing acne, diabetes, or cancer, or simply losing excess weight and gaining more energy. People who do the programs are held accountable for achieving their goals and get to experience powerful results. The Earth Diet is free for everyone to do, but these programs are for people who want to commit to this lifestyle fully and want to have a health coach with them to guide them at every step. We teach you all the tools you need to live a powerful natural lifestyle that you love. We look at the toxicities in your lifestyle and make a strategy with you to incorporate more nature one step at a time.

**CHECK OUT WWW.THEEARTHDIET.COM/ PACKAGES FOR EARTH DIET PACKAGES AND GIFT BOXES!**

By the time this book comes out, there may be additional companies and people you would be interested in becoming aware of. So always visit the resources page on my website, TheEarthDiet.com/resources, for the most current information and up-to-date offers and discounts from my friends and partners.

## ENDNOTES

## Part I: Why the Earth Diet?

### CHAPTER 1: THE EARTH DIET BASICS

1. John Andrews, "Why a Microwave Oven Is Bad for Your Health," NaturalNews.com (September 6, 2007). http://www.naturalnews.com/022015_microwave_oven_power.html.

2. Thierry Vrain, Ph.D., "Former Pro-GMO Scientist Speaks Out on the Real Dangers of Genetically Engineered Food," FoodRevolution.org (May 11, 2013). http://www.foodrevolution.org/blog/former-pro-gmo-scientist.

3. Wayne Dyer as cited by TinyBuddha.com.

4. Mark David, M.D., *The Slow Down Diet: Eating for Pleasure, Energy, and Weight Loss* (Rochester, VT: Healing Arts Press, 2005), 105.

5. Ibid.: 106.

### CHAPTER 2: SELF-HEALING WITH THE EARTH DIET

1. To read the official definition of the term *organic*, as it applies to food industry regulations in the United States, visit the website of the National Organic Program of the U.S. Department of Agriculture: http://www.ams.usda.gov/AMSv1.0/nop.

2. To find out more about T. Colin Campbell's research, visit the website of his foundation: http://tcolincampbell.org.

3. T. Colin Campbell, Ph.D., *The China Study* (Dallas, TX: BenBella Books, 2005), 3.

4. Jack Kornfield, *Buddha's Little Instruction Book* (New York: Bantam Books, 1994), 47.

5. Norman Cousins, *The Anatomy of an Illness* (New York: W. W. Norton & Company, 1979), 63.

6. Bruce H. Lipton, Ph.D., *The Biology of Belief* (Carlsbad, CA: Hay House, 2008), xxvi.

7. Wayne Dyer as cited by Entheos.com.

### CHAPTER 3: THE EARTH DIET LIFESTYLE

1. Andrew Weil, M.D., *Spontaneous Healing* (New York: Alfred A. Knopf, 1995), 134–35.

2. Louise Hay, *Love Your Body, Expanded Edition* (Carlsbad, CA: Hay House, 1989).

### CHAPTER 4: PREPARATIONS

1. "Frequently Asked Questions," GersonInstitute.org. http://gerson.org/gerpress/faqs-diet.

2. "Non-Stick Cookware Continues to Prove Its Toxicity," Mercola.com. http://articles.mercola.com/sites/articles/archive/2008/03/06/non-stick-cookware-continues-to-prove-its-toxicity.aspx. Also, Fiona Haynes, "Is Nonstick Cookware Safe?" About.com (accessed August 8, 2013). http://lowfatcooking.about.com/od/healthandfitness/a/nonstickpans.htm.

## CHAPTER 6: YOUR FIRST STEPS

1. ThinkExist.com.

2. Very little is known about Hippocrates, the "father of medicine," who lived in Greece during the fifth century B.C.E. Many insights on health, such as this one, were attributed to him by his followers and their descendants. Contemporary doctors upon graduation from medical school swear an oath that bears his name.

# INDEX

# "Believe you can and you're halfway there."

— Theodore Roosevelt

I am grateful to Stacey Smith at Hay House for introducing me to publisher Reid Tracy, who has invested his faith, trust, and support in me and this project. Louise Hay is such an inspiration. Her meditations and affirmations helped me during the writing of this book. Also among the Hay House family, I am thankful for having worked with Patricia Gift, Editor Jessica Kelley, Richelle Zizian, Shannon Littrell, Christy Salinas, Shannon Godwin, Ellen Scordato, Michelle Ocampo, and Johanne Mahaffey.

Thank you to Stephanie Gunning, my publishing consultant, for how fun and easy you made the writing process. It was great working side by side with you in New York City, juicing and eating fresh cucumber and raw chocolate.

Thank you to the team who photographed the Earth Diet recipes and made them come to life and even used organic ingredients for the photo shoot! You did an incredible job: Ellen Scordato, Michele Jerry, Allen Owens, Dave Ruben Lewis, Alyssa Alia, and Geovanna Kurdek.

Thank you to my publicist Ashley Sanburg for helping get the word out about this transformative natural lifestyle! Roxxe Ireland, thank you for your superb photographs of me and my food. You're an artist.

Thank you Howard Hoffman for your mentorship and for providing me with daily alkalizing greens drinks that kept me so refreshed and focused during this entire process. Having you as part of the team makes a huge difference! And thank you to the Phresh Products team, especially Matt, Donna, and Jeff Stuchala. Dr. Leonard Coldwell has been so generous with me, a real fountain of resources and insights on what would be important to include in the book. Dr. C, I want you to know how much I value your friendship and mentorship. Thank you Noah Loin of Noah's Rock'n Raw Chocolates for making sure I had plenty of delicious, raw, healthy chocolate while working on this book! It kept me excited. Thank you, Briony, the founder of ADORN, and the rest of the team in Australia, for providing me with plant-based, animal-cruelty-free makeup for the photo shoot and events while promoting this book.

I cherish my mother, Vicki Gray, and appreciate being her daughter. She was the first to teach me about natural foods and gardening. Mum, thank you for inspiring me to create the now-famous Raw Cashew Cheesecake! I am grateful also to my father, Bernard Werner, who taught me about sustainable living and how to be resourceful with solar energy and rainwater collection. Their interests have made a deep and positive impact on my beliefs and attitudes. To my sisters, Nadine and Caitlin: I appreciate your love and how you inspire me, as sisters should! Nadine, I put the Hummus recipe in this book for you! Aunt Tammy and Uncle Michael and Cousin Bernie: You are my rock-solid support system. Nanna, I love you. You make me smile. Thank you, Rock, for teaching me how to be a disciplined worker.

I would like to thank the Aboriginal community of Alice Springs, Australia, for instilling in me the belief from an early age that it was possible to live off the land and in harmony with the earth. I was fortunate to attend Gillen Primary School, whose staff took me on excursions camping in the Bush, where I was introduced to the indigenous elders who taught us how to survive. My classmates and I learned how to survive by finding our own food and water. At Gillen I was nurtured—especially by my grade four teacher, Miss Thompson—to understand that I could do anything I set my mind to. She empowered me with a self-confidence that gave me the foundation needed to start my business.

Many people helped me find my way back to health. I am grateful to my early blog readers, who helped me stay accountable when I quit eating junk food and transformed my lifestyle. Thank you, Carol Lucas, for expressing your faith in me in tangible ways. Your support means the world to me. To the current readers of The Earth Diet blog, you inspire me to keep going. You are honest, curious, and generous. It is my pleasure to serve you every day.

To my Earth Diet team, thank you. Salvatore Fiteni, thank you for your persistence, good ideas, and big heart. Laura Lipari, nutritional analyst, thank you for calculating the nutrient content of my recipes. Earth Diet health coaches, Chizelle Sharon, Patrick Vahey, Emily Rose Shaw, and Jessie Jean, you are helping so many people get healthy with the Earth Diet one-on-one nutritional counseling programs. I couldn't spread the message of the Earth Diet without you guys. Thank you Debra Toomey for being such a great client and so willing to transform. Your blog earthdietblogs.com/DebbieSavesHerLife is so inspiring. Thank you for making me a better health coach. Thank you to my wonderful distributor Mark Darougar and Robert from Health by Design.

Thank you Brandon Redlinger for your marketing direction with this book launch. Thank you Christopher Schrack of LW Films. Thank you Derek for your faith and support.

I'd like to acknowledge Demetra and Eleni Simos for having faith in me from the beginning, Paul Riedel of Big Al's Family Fitness in Amityville, New York; especially Craig Margulies of Organic Corner in Massapequa, New York, and the rest of the team at OC: Rowan, Greg, Jackie, Heather, and Jasmine; Kathy from the Water Well in Huntington, NY; Jody Loin and Elizabeth Garden—thank you for your expert gardening tips; Dr. Thomas Ianniello of the North Isle Wellness Center in Miller Place, New York; Jean Weiss and her Wellness Home—would not have done this without your support; Lynnette Pate; Mike Adams of Natural News; Robert Scott Bell of NaturalNews Radio; the Roth family; and Heather Dean—I value you so much! Thank you for believing in me.

A special thanks to Eckhart Tolle: Listening to your inspirational audio recordings helped me stay motivated and feeling relaxed and empowered while I was producing this book. I am grateful for the life of Nelson Mandela. From his writing, I learned courage, gratitude, patience, and being unreasonable. During my healing journey, his story kept me going in the direction my heart was leading. Thank you to Gandhi for leaving a powerful legacy and for reminding me to be the change, which made me realize that if I want to live on a healthier planet, I need to be healthy and make the healthiest choices possible.

Thank you to other people that I have worked with after writing these acknowledgments.

Thank you to every person reading this book, and every person I have ever met that has helped me grow to be who I am today.

# ABOUT THE AUTHOR

**LIANA WERNER-GRAY** is an advocate for natural healing using a healthy diet and lifestyle. After healing herself of many health conditions through embracing a natural lifestyle, she began lecturing and teaching about the Earth Diet internationally. Liana teaches raw food and cooking classes around the world and has fed many people good-tasting, healthy foods and drinks.

Liana is the founder and owner of The Earth Diet Inc., where she helps people all over the world find recipes that work for them. Through her company, she has helped thousands of people improve, and in some cases even entirely heal, conditions such as acne, addictions, cancer, diabetes, depression, heart disease, obesity, and more.

Liana was born and raised in Australia. In her final year of schooling she received the school's award for the arts, the Liana Nappi Award. She was named Miss Earth Australia in 2009 by People's Choice, the third-largest beauty pageant in the world. During the same competition, she was also awarded Best in Environmental Speech, Green Achievers, and the Innovators award.

Liana has starred in films that received international praise and awards. She continues to work in the entertainment business, as well as promoting a healthy lifestyle. Her intention is to live her life the best she can, and hopefully inspire others to live the lives of their dreams through a healthy lifestyle. She currently lives in New York City.

**WEBSITE:** lianawernergray.com